Stefano Fanti – Mohsen Farsad – Luigi Mansi

Atlas of PET / CT

A Quick Guide to Image Interpretation

Stefano Fanti – Mohsen Farsad – Luigi Mansi

Atlas of PET / CT
A Quick Guide to
Image Interpretation

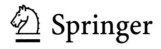 Springer

Stefano Fanti, Prof.
Director of PET
University of Bologna
40100 Bologna
Italy
stefano.fanti@aosp.bo.it

Luigi Mansi, Prof.
Chairman and Director of Nuclear Medicine
Second University of Naples
80129 Naples
Italy
luigi.mansi@unina2.it

Mohsen Farsad, Dr.
Assistant Director of Nuclear Medicine
Central Hospital of Bolzano
39100 Bolzano
Italy
mohsen.farsad@asbz.it

ISBN 978-3-540-77771-7   e-ISBN 978-3-540-77772-4

DOI 10.1007/978-3-540-77772-4

Library of Congress Control Number: 2008940062

© 2009 Springer-Verlag Berlin Heidelberg

Cover design: Frido Steinen-Broo, eStudio Calamar, Spain
Production & Typesetting: le-tex publishing services oHG, Leipzig, Germany

Printed on acid-free paper

9 8 7 6 5 4 3 2 1

springer.com

Acknowledgements

The realization of this project has involved so many people that it is difficult to know where to begin saying thank you, and we are likely to miss someone out.

The authors are grateful to Prof. Fabrizio Calliada for writing the chapter on the radiologist's perspective.

Stefano Fanti would like to thank all his colleagues, in particular Dr. Vincenzo Allegri, Dr. Margherita Maffione, and Dr. GianCarlo Montini for their collaboration in the selection of cases, Prof. Nino Monetti and Dr. Roberto Franchi for their mentorship, and Dr. Paolo Castellucci and Dr. Cristina Nanni for their invaluable professionalism and friendship.

Mohsen Farsad would like to thank Dr. Luzian Osele for his constructive suggestions, Dr. Patrizia Pernter for her technical advice and criticism in the preparation of this book, and Dr. Adil Al-Nahhas and all the colleagues in Bologna for introducing him to PET imaging.

Luigi Mansi would like to acknowledge Dr. Vincenzo Cuccurullo, Dr. Pier Francesco Rambaldi, and all the students who greatly stimulated a growth in knowledge based on a productive dialectic discussion. Of his teachers, he would like to thank Prof. Marco Salvatore, and revive the memory of Prof. Salvatore Venuta, who introduced him to the study of deoxy-glucose and thymidine in oncology in 1975, and that of Dr. Giovanni Di Chiro, who permitted him to participate as a pioneer of PET-FDG development in the early 1980s. Lastly, he would like to dedicate this book to his son, Elvio David, hoping to transfer to him a lifelong passion for learning.

Contents

Chapter 1 Normal Distribution of FDG

Normal Distribution of FDG

Today, more than 95% of PET procedures worldwide are performed with F-18 fluoro-deoxyglucose (FDG). This situation is dependent at first by practical reasons: Fluorine 18 is one of the four most important positron emitters, easily produced by "standard" cyclotrons, with the capability to radiolabel relevant biological molecules. Because of the favorable half-life (110 minutes) with respect to shorter-lived C-11, N-13 and O-15, Fluorine-18 is the only one in this series that can be distributed also to PET centers without cyclotrons. Therefore, it can be used in a wider geographic area covering, in more developed countries, all the national territory.

From a chemical point of view, Fluorine is a halogen allowing a very stable binding that does not affect the functional part of the molecule. But the real "absolute" value of F-18 is derived by its capability to radiolabel deoxy-glucose producing FDG; i. e., the glucose's tracer. Glucose is an essential compound for living organisms, being the most important carbon supplier in energy producing metabolic processes depending largely on its availability.

Pathophysiology of Glucose and FDG's Biodistribution

For a correct reading of PET-FDG images, based on the interpretation of all molecular involved events, we have to first analyze the normal glucose distribution, starting from the knowledge of its pathophysiological behavior. Devoting to more extensive and/or specialized publications a deeper analysis of FDG as a "molecular tracer" of glucose transporters (six isoforms: GLUT 1 to GLUT 5 and GLUT 7 have been identified so far), it is important to remember that the glucose uptake in human cells can take place through two mechanisms: facilitated diffusion and active transport.

The first one is a carrier-mediated transport, therefore characterized by saturation (and influenced by insulin, increasing its rate up to 20-fold). It means that a competitive inhibition of transport can occur in the presence of a second ligand that binds to the same carrier. This explains the strong interference on FDG uptake determined by diabetes and, more in general, by variations in glucose and insulin levels in the blood. For these reasons, to standardize the analysis of FDG distribution it is crucial to define a fasting time (at least 4–6

hours), a serum glucose range and, in diabetes, the timing after insulin injection. Although chronic hyperglycemia is less disturbing with respect to the acute variety, PET scans are preferably performed with serum glucose levels in the range of 70–110 ng/dl. It is better to avoid examinations in patients with glucose levels higher than 200 ng/dl or in the presence of hyperinsulinemia, both of which reduce diagnostic accuracy because of their strong interference on biodistribution.

Being less diffuse, glucose's active transport, occurring against an electrochemical gradient, functions only in certain special epithelial cells specifically adapted for active absorption, such as those present in gastrointestinal membranes or through the renal tubules.

FDG "Trapping"

The biochemical fates of glucose start with phosphorylation, immediately after its entrance in cells. The phosphorylation, both for glucose and FDG, is promoted by hexokinase in the large majority of cells, being dependent by glucokinase in the liver. After this first step, glucose-6-phosphate progresses in its metabolic fate, after a dephosphorylation mediated by glucose-6-phosphatase, undergoing glycolysis (and/or to the storage of glycogen and/or to lipids or proteins conversion). Conversely, FDG-6-phosphate is not further metabolized in the glycolytic pathway, remaining "intracellularly trapped", because of the lack of significant amounts of FDG-6-phosphatase to reverse the phosphorylation. This is a "major advantage" for PET-FDG imaging: while the radiolabeled "native" glucose has a metabolism that is too fast to easily permit a PET study, the "trapped" FDG can reliably "in vivo" trace glucose concentration, reflecting the glucose metabolism in the whole organism, except for kidneys.

At this level, while normal individuals do not excrete glucose trough the urinary system, an intense FDG uptake is observed in kidneys, ureters and bladders. In fact, whereas normal glucose is freely filtered by glomeruli and rapidly reabsorbed by the nephron, FDG is poorly reabsorbed after filtration, being excreted in a large amount in the urine. Other F-18 labeled radiochemical forms, derived from FDG's catabolism, can further explain radioactivity in the urinary system.

It has to be pointed out that, in individuals with normal renal function, 50% of the radioactivity reaches the bladder at two hours. This is a major advantage in reducing radiation dosimetry because of the consequent low effective half-life. Conversely, to define a major contraindication, it has to be remembered that FDG cross the placenta, being distributed mainly in fetal brains and excreted by fetal kidneys. Breastfeeding is contraindicated before 10 hours after i.v. injection of FDG.

Physiological and Para-Physiological Distribution of FDG

Devoting the knowledge of more precise rules and technical issues to national and/or international protocols, we will briefly describe here the standard procedure as a premise to the normal whole body FDG pattern.

The patient is i.v. injected, after fasting for at least 4–6 hours, but while well-hydrated. During the injection and the following uptake phase preceding the scan, the individual has to be at rest in a quiet room, comfortable and relaxed. In particular, he has to try to avoid such actions as chewing, eating, running and any other exercise and/or sensory activation affecting FDG distribution, mainly increasing muscular or regional cerebral uptake. Since it is impossible to avoid swallowing, it has to be remembered, mainly for patients undergoing a PET scan for head and neck tumors, the effect on the FDG's uptake in the vocal cords when talking.

Under standard conditions the highest FDG activity is seen at the cerebral level (mainly in gray matter), since the brain is the only organ exclusively using glucose as a carburant. At fast, cardiac uptake (left ventricle) is variable, but most frequently mild and homogeneous. Occasionally, a difficult analysis can be determined by a high blood pool activity at the level of the great vessels, mainly in mediastinum. While liver and spleen show low-grade diffuse activity, variable uptake is seen in the gastrointestinal system, sometimes creating difficulties in the analysis and problems in differential diagnosis. This activity can be related both to smooth muscle uptake as well as to the intra-luminal content. Low and/ or absent concentration is observed at the level of bone marrow. Similarly, no activity is seen at the level of normal lymph nodes, but after FDG's extravasation at the injection site, determining high focal uptake in the draining regional glands. Moderate activity can be seen in tonsils, salivary glands, myelohyoid muscles and, in young patients, in the thymus, adenoidal tissue and testicles. No uptake is normally seen at the level of lungs, since a slight activity in posterior and inferior segments is sometimes present. The skeletal muscle's uptake, being low at rest, increases as a specific response to stress and/ or exercise in the involved muscular cells. An increased uptake can be determined by many conditions such as hyperventilation, hiccuping, torticollis and intense eye movement, as a result of involuntary tensions. The muscular uptake is generally bilateral and symmetric. Conversely, an apparent unilateral pathological concentration can be observed contralaterally to a nerve palsy. The urinary excretion, determining a high normal background at the renal and vesicle level, can create difficulties in evaluating FDG's pathological uptake mainly in kidneys and prostates. Small areas of ureteric stasis may simulate lymphadenopathy. The presence of anomalous locations of kidneys and ureters has to be known so as to avoid mistakes in PET images interpretation. Thyroid uptake can be occasionally observed in clinically normal patients, being more frequently caused by thyroiditis or hyperthyroidism. In premenopausal women (and/ or in women taking estrogens) breast tissue often demonstrates moderate symmetrical FDG concentration. Intense uptake is presented by breastfeeding mothers. A faint-to-moderate uterine uptake can be observed during menstruation. In adipose tissue a typical symmetric intense uptake can be determined by active brown fat, mainly in winter months in patients with a lower body mass index.

Since the lesion's detectability in nuclear medicine is dependent on lesion/background ratio, it is evident that major difficulties in PET-FDG are present at the cerebral level and/or in the abdominal-pelvic territory, where activities deriving from the gastrointestinal and urinary emunctories can disturb.

Nevertheless, many physiological and para-physiological uptakes can be easily distinguished by the morphostructural information obtained by CT. To avoid problems, some authors also suggest the administration of muscle relaxants, cleansing bowel preparations and the placement of a Foley's catheter. However, because of difficulties in standardizing these procedures and of the impossibility of reliably avoiding possible pitfalls, a "keep it simple" strategy is more frequently adopted.

Pathophysiology of FDG Uptake in Cancer (and Benign Diseases)

Cancer cells are generally characterized by an increased glucose metabolism with respect to normal cells. In particular, malignancy is frequently associated with the appearance of new phenotypes with a higher expression of glucose transporters, an increasing rate of cell proliferation, protein and DNA synthesis, and anarchic neo-angiogenesis. All these conditions determine a significant increase of glucose's uptake, to provide the fuel necessary to answer new requests for energy, produced mainly through anaerobic glycolysis. FDG uptake and bio-distribution in tumors is therefore influenced by many parameters, such as increased glucose turnover, expression of glucose transporters and hexokinase activity, being also dependent (through non-specific mechanisms, independent of the neoplastic transformation) on the increased number of cell divisions. Devoting a deeper analysis of molecular mechanisms to wider and/or specialized publications, and not being interesting for the purposes of this Atlas to discuss pathophysiological premises to clinical indications in cardiology and neurology, we define here some general behaviors and provide suggestions helpful in the analysis of PET-FDG images in oncology and other benign diseases to be taken into account for differential diagnosis:

A. FDG Uptake in Tumors

- The large majority of malignant tumors show an increased FDG uptake.
- FDG's uptake is influenced by the "biological malignancy", i.e. by issues such as growth rate, hypoxia, histopathology concerning both the histotype and grading. Intense uptake is more frequently observed in lymphoma, melanoma, colorectal, esophageal and head/neck cancer, NSCLC, sarcoma and, more in general, in high grade tumors.
- A minority of tumors can present low or absent FDG uptake. This pattern is mainly dependent on differentiation, as evidenced by the absence of FDG uptake in the large majority of lesions in patients with well-differentiated thyroid carcinoma or neuroendocrine tumors (NET). Low and/or absent FDG uptake is also frequently seen in low-grade hepatocarcinoma, also because of the presence of a higher glucose-6-phosphatase activity resulting in a low FDG uptake, in tumors characterized by a low growth rate, as in prostate cancer, in tumors characterized by functional features as the mucinous production, or by a particular tumor morphology, as can be observed in primary ovarian cancer, frequently consisting of large cystic portions.

B. FDG Uptake as Prognostic Indicator

- In tumors with a higher prevalence of normally not concentrating lesions, such as NET, thyroid or liver carcinomas, FDG concentration defines a worse prognosis with respect to patients not showing uptake.
- Similarly, in a very large majority of tumors, including in a single category all the patients bearing the same histotype, a higher uptake indicates a worse fate.

In fact, it has been demonstrated that FDG uptake in cancer tissue is determined, among other factors, by tumor proliferation rates, aggressiveness and rate of neo-angiogenesis. This relationship, however, is non-linear, mainly in rapidly growing tumors, since it is dependent on many parameters, including the various percentages of anaerobic metabolism and the presence of necrosis.

C. FDG Uptake as Recurrence Identificator

- Recurrent disease, because of the loss of differentiated features, is in general characterized by a higher FDG uptake with respect to the primary tumor.
- There is no FDG uptake in the absence of viable cancer cells and therefore in necrosis and/or fibrosis.
- In cancer patients, when a FDG uptake is observed at diagnosis and/or at the pre-therapeutic control, a negative PET scan at follow up can reliably exclude recurrence with respect to post-therapeutic fibrosis and/or necrosis.
- The opposite, however, is never true; i.e., FDG uptake is not necessarily determined by recurrence, because of possible false positive results (see below).

D. FDG Uptake as Guide to Biopsy and/or to Define the Target in Radiotherapy

- In inhomogeneous tumors, FDG uptake is higher in the most malignant part of the lesion, being lower in the most differentiated components and absent in necrotic or fibrotic areas.
- PET-FDG can guide a biopsy to the most malignant part of the tumor.
- For the same reason, PET-FDG allows a better definition of the "biological target" in radiotherapy. PET-CT images can serve to design a tailored therapeutic plan, giving a higher dosage to the most malignant part of the tumor, and reducing radiation to normal tissues.

E. FDG Uptake Variation as a Marker of Response to Therapy

- Glucose uptake rapidly decreases after an effective therapeutic action, remaining unchanged and/or increasing in non-responders. Therefore, FDG's uptake can be an early marker of the therapeutic response in tumors with respect to the information allowed by CT, US and MRI detecting late variations on size and structure; moreover, it is less reliably connected to the therapeutic efficacy. This FDG advantage has already been demonstrated in many patients subjected to chemotherapy. A wider and deeper experience on the possible clinical usefulness in oncology, including all histotypes, better defining timing of evaluation and capability to also predict the response to radiotherapy, is under evaluation

F. False Positive Results Due to FDG Uptake in Benign Diseases

- The highest percentage of benign lesions do not present FDG uptake, and are therefore distinguishable from malignant ones in the large majority of cases.
- A minority of benign lesions can show FDG uptake, generally with a lower entity with respect to malignant tumors.
- FDG accumulates in activated white cells and macrophages. Therefore, it can be concentrated at the level of active inflammatory processes either infectious or non-infectious.
- The presence of false positive results can create problems in diagnosis (and staging), but is less critical in re-staging and at follow up.
- It is necessary to be very careful in utilizing PET-FDG for a primary diagnosis, mainly in patients with a high prevalence of inflammatory or granulomatous conditions (tuberculosis, sarcoidosis, etc.).
- FDG uptake can be present at the level of the wound healing (in general up to 6 months), in the inflammatory reaction after radiotherapy, in associated benign lymphadenopathy or infections, in lung atelectasis and pleural effusion and in reactive thymus hyperplasia (sometimes appearing in young patients after chemotherapy). Dubious images can also be due to pathological conditions such as gastritis, gastroesophageal reflux, diverticulitis, inflammatory bowel disease, abscess, hiatal hernia and benign uterine fibroids. The uptake determined by benign healing fractures or arthropathies can be critical to avoiding possible mistakes in diagnosing bone metastases. A diffuse increase at the level of bone marrow (and/or of spleen) can be observed after the administration of granulocyte colony stimulating factor.

G. Usefulness of FDG in Benign Diseases

- Without discussing here the clinical usefulness in cardiology and in neuropsychiatry, and putting in evidence that false positive results in oncology occurs in only a very low percentage of the PET results, it has to be pointed out that, although it may have possible negative effects on specificity in patients with cancer, FDG uptake can also determine useful clinical indications in benign diseases.
- For example, PET-FDG is a first line procedure in the diagnosis of fever of unknown origin (FUO), because of the need for the highest sensitivity to detect occult lesions, not negatively counterbalanced by a reduced specificity. Other useful information can be obtained in defining the activity in many inflammatory diseases, to detect activated atherosclerotic plaques in great vessels, to determine the presence of a reaction in the area surrounding prosthetic devices, and in autoimmune diseases, etc.

H. Differential Diagnosis Using PET-FDG in Oncology

- Role of quantitation. To increase information acquired through visual analysis, quantitative and/or semi-quantitative methods can be utilized. This evaluation is outside the scope of our publication. Although precise and rigorous quantitative procedures have been proposed, the only one used today in the clinical routine is the so-called SUV.
- Standardized uptake value (SUV). This is a semi-quantitative method, defining the FDG uptake's entity based on a ratio approximately referring the lesion value to the whole body activity. It is affected by many parameters, such as serum glucose level, body weight and compartmental glucose distribution. For these reasons it can not be considered an absolutely reliable method. Nevertheless, it can have a useful clinical role, complementary with visual analysis, mainly for determining temporal variations in the same patient, and therefore the effect of a therapy. SUV has also been proposed for helping differential diagnosis in solitary pulmonary nodules through the definition of an uptake threshold (for lesions higher than 1 cm, cancer is more probable in the presence of a SUV higher than 2.5).

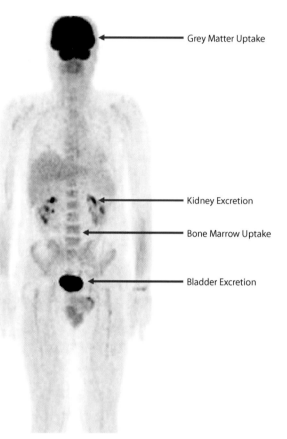

Grey Matter Uptake

Kidney Excretion

Bone Marrow Uptake

Bladder Excretion

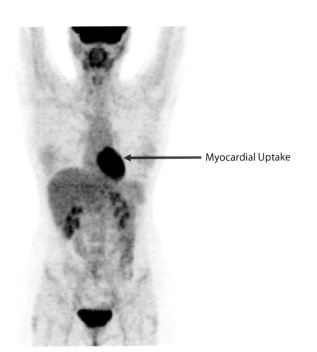

Myocardial Uptake

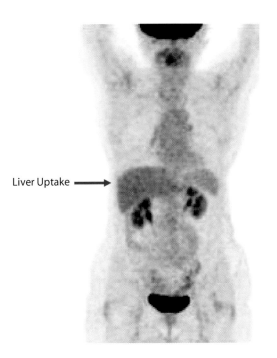

Liver Uptake

Teaching point

Myocardial uptake is quite unpredictable, as related to several factors, probably the most important being fasting.

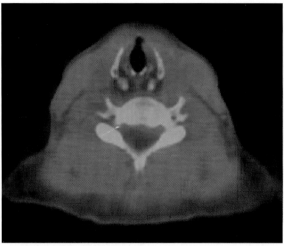 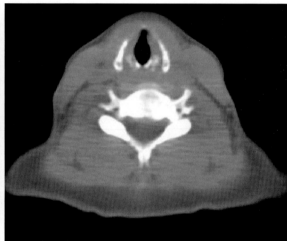

◘ Cricoarytenoid muscles

Teaching point

Muscles usually do not avidly uptake FDG, assuming that fasting has been respected and that intense contraction has not occurred during the uptake period (especially during the first 20 minutes after FDG injection). However, it may be difficult to prevent patients from talking and swallowing, therefore some uptake in the head and neck muscle has to be expected.

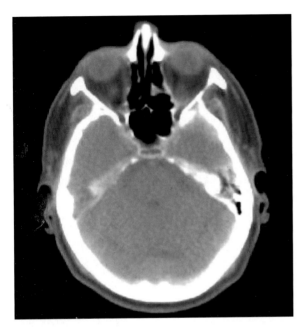 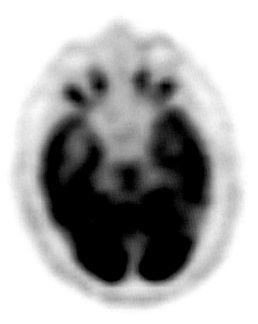

🔹 Ocular muscles FDG uptake

Teaching point

To avoid muscle uptake it is mandatory to have the patient at rest for at least 20 minutes after injection; also administration of myorelaxant has been suggested. With the use of PET-CT fused images it is usually possible to distinguish muscle uptake from pathologic findings.

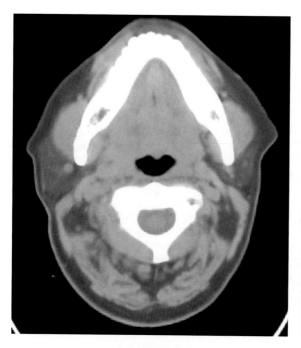
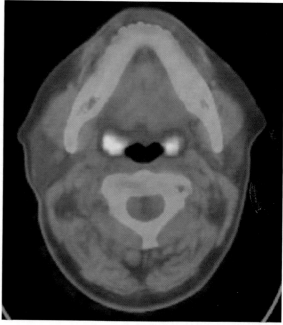

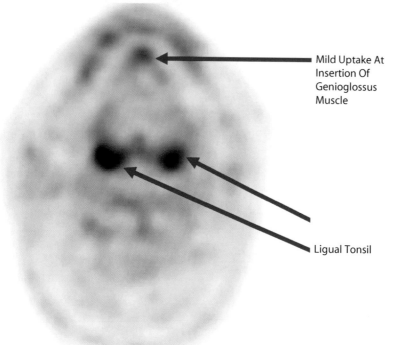

Mild Uptake At Insertion Of Genioglossus Muscle

Ligual Tonsil

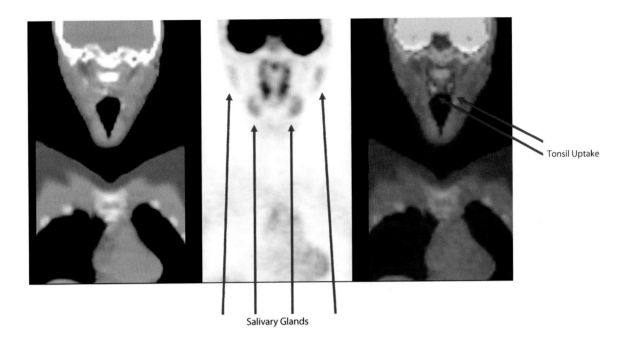

Tonsil Uptake

Salivary Glands

Teaching point

Salivary glands and lymphatic tissue can show a variable degree of FDG uptake; this has to be taken into particular account in diseases affecting these organs.

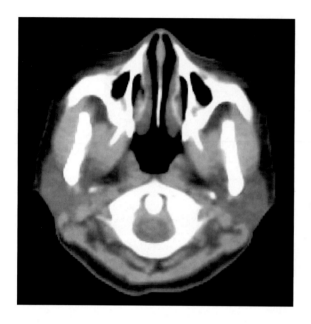
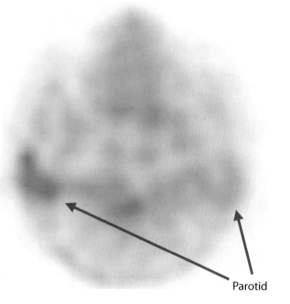

Parotid

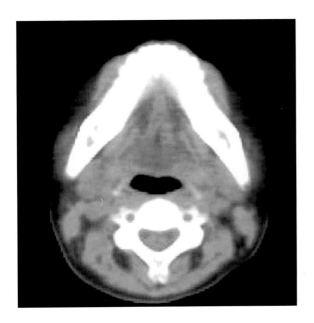

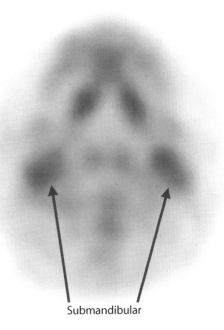

Submandibular

Teaching point

Usually physiologic uptake in the salivary glands is symmetric, but not necessarily in all cases and glands. Again, PET-CT fusion images are extremely helpful to establish the site of uptake.

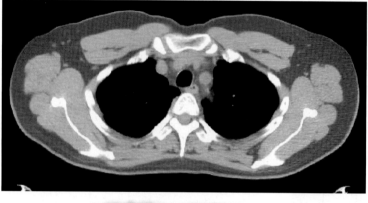

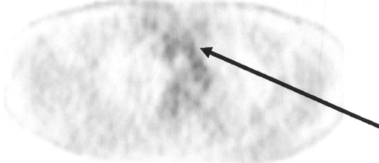

Blood Pool
Activity of
Great Vessels

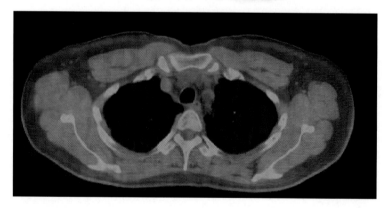

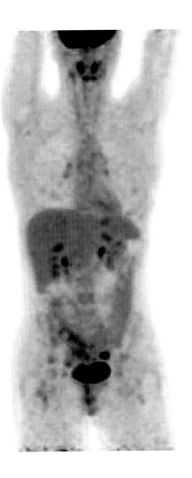

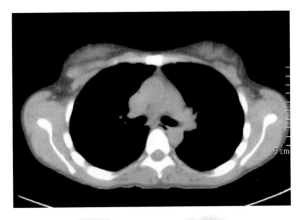

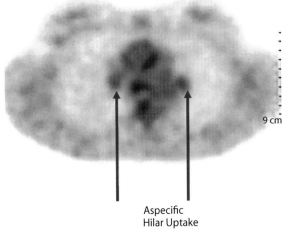

Aspecific
Hilar Uptake

Teaching point

Non-specific uptake at both lung hila can be observed quite frequently, maybe related with aspecific inflammation. It has to be taken into particular consideration in order to avoid a wrong report: it is usually not intense and symmetrical.

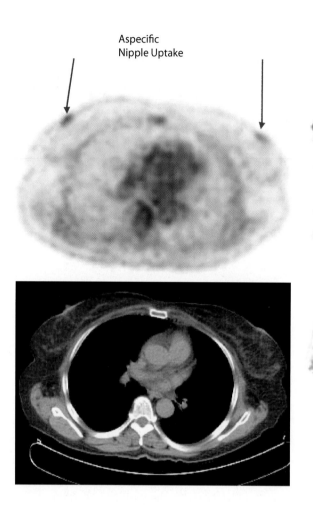

Aspecific
Nipple Uptake

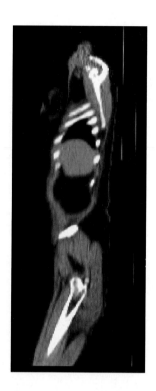

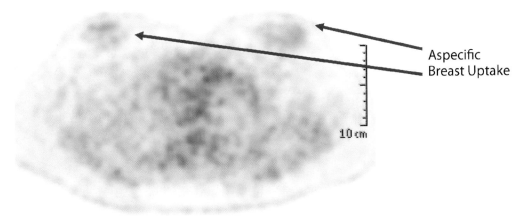

Aspecific
Breast Uptake

10 cm

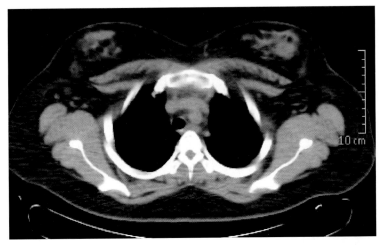

10 cm

Teaching point

Breast and nipples frequently show a
faint uptake. It should be considered
physiological, given that no focal area of
intense uptake is observed.

17

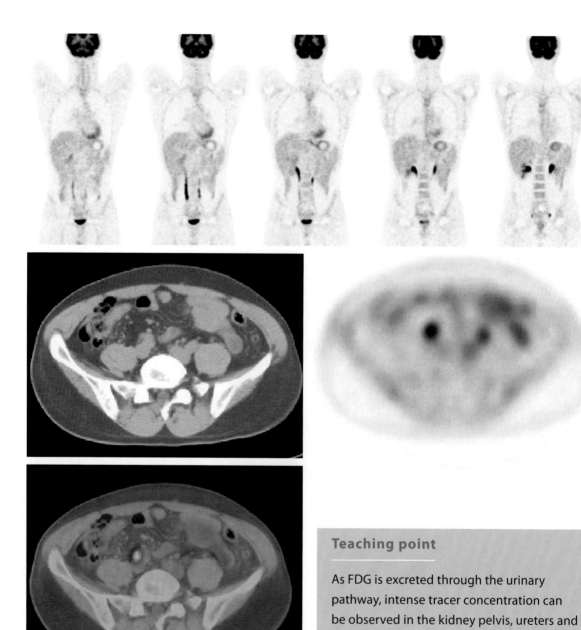

Teaching point

As FDG is excreted through the urinary pathway, intense tracer concentration can be observed in the kidney pelvis, ureters and bladder.

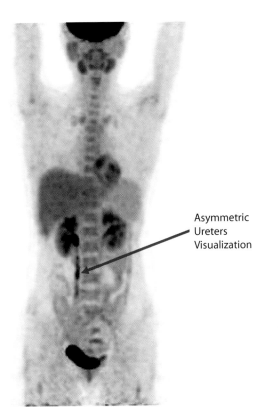

Asymmetric
Ureters
Visualization

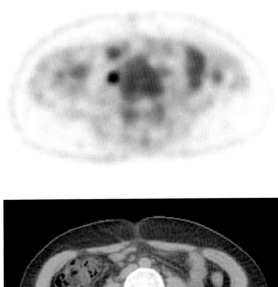

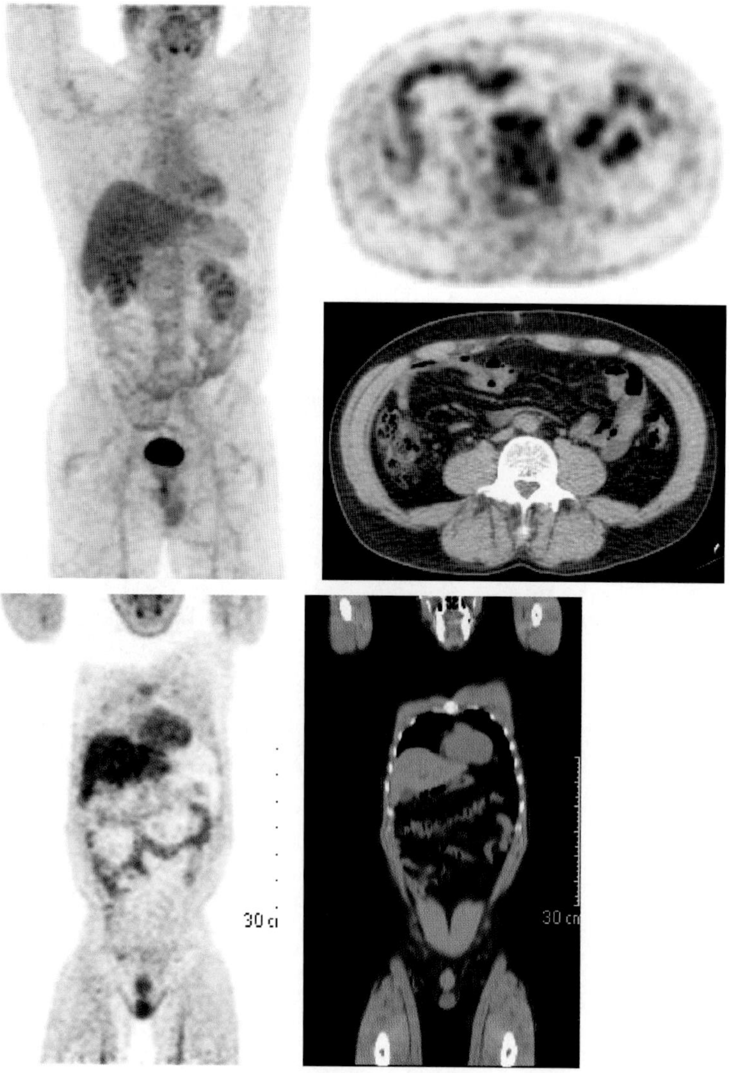

■ Aspecific bowel FDG uptake

Teaching point

FDG uptake is frequently observed at bowel level; again the use of PET-CT fused images is important to correctly identify the site of uptake.

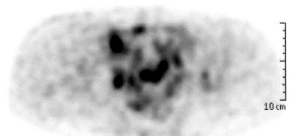

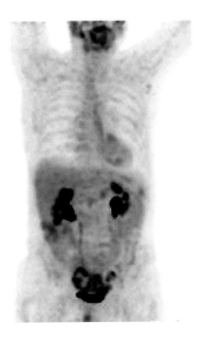

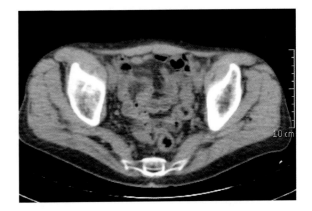

◘ Aspecific bowel FDG uptake

Teaching point

The degree of FDG uptake at bowel level is almost unpredictable, and a quite intense uptake can be seen, especially at cecal and sigma level. The use of PET-CT fused images is important to correctly identify the site of uptake, and in cases of focal intense uptake, referring the patient for further evaluation has to be suggested.

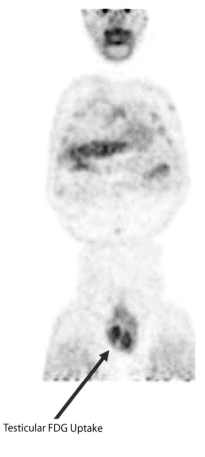

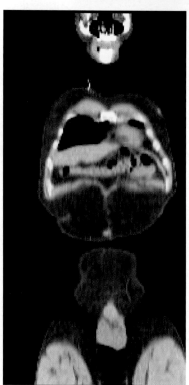

Testicular FDG Uptake

Teaching point

The testis almost always show a faint FDG uptake; in young patients the degree of uptake can be more relevant.

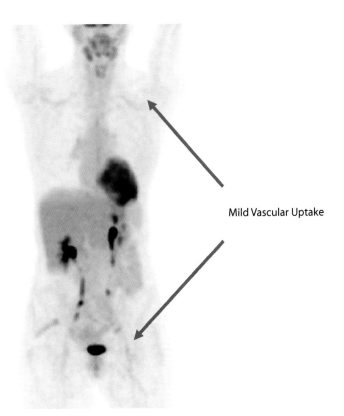

Mild Vascular Uptake

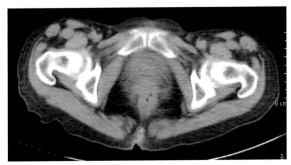

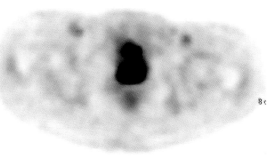

Teaching point

Blood vessels may show faint uptake.
It should be considered physiological,
especially in older patients.

Chapter 2   Contrast-Enhanced CT in PET-CT (PET-CECT)

PET-CT: The Radiologist Point of View

The CT part of the combined PET-CT imaging requires some facts that "Nucs" doctors need to know about CT technology and CT contrast media.

The choice of slice number should really be considered a "non problem" matter in an oncologic field. Even an old and simple 4 slices CT is able to perform a whole body examination in an acceptable time, allowing the study of every portion of the body within an appropriate timeframe. Increasing the number of the slices reduces, of course, the examination time, but the diagnostic improvement is especially evident in vascular studies, and 64 or more slices are really mandatory only for cardiac studies. For that reason, 8 or 16 slices machines should be considered absolutely adequate if heart studies are not planned.

To perform a correct diagnostic CT examination it is necessary to know more than something about contrast agents. Essentially there are two different kinds of contrast: **oral contrast and intravenous contrast**.

Oral contrast: if your CT experience is outperforming, oral contrast is probably unnecessary, but otherwise oral contrast allows one to easily distinguish bowel loops from lymph nodes or other normal and abnormal abdominal structures. It is possible to choose between positive or neutral endoluminal contrast agents. Positive contrasts are barium sulphate, 1.5 g/100 ml–1000 cc; and meglumine diatrizoate, 3%–1000 cc. Positive contrast agents allow better delineation of gastrointestinal tract organs from their surrounding structures but exhibit potential PET attenuation artifacts. Neutral oral contrasts are water or low-density barium sulfate suspension; they are less evident than positive contrast agent but exhibit some important advantages: better delineation of the gastrointestinal tract mucosa and i.v. contrast mucosal enhancement (normally obscured by positive oral contrast), without potential PET/CT attenuation artifacts. Which neutral contrast would be more useful? Water is cheap, but absorbed quickly and is only good for stomach and proximal small bowel. Low-density barium sulfate suspension is more expensive, but allows better distension of small/large bowel.

Intravenous (i.v.) contrast agents allow better anatomic detail, delineate vascular structures and improve overall CT contrast with increased diagnostic accuracy and confidence. Iodine is a temporal and spatial variable introduced in the vascular circulation, allowing better physiological evaluation of the entire body, allowing one to study tissue enhancement patterns with improved diagnostic accuracy and confidence, especially in tumors with only mild or no increase in 18F-FDG uptake by supporting lesion detection and characterization. You don't need to perform a separate "diagnostic" CECT scan with reduced radiation dose to the patient. Intravenous iodine contrast agents are different in concentration and iodine content so you need to review protocol studies beforehand, as there are multiple options. Iodine concentration is variable from 200 to 400 mg/mL. Higher concentrations (350–400) are suitable for abdominal (especially liver) or vascular studies; lower concentrations (300) are used in lung parenchymal studies. Specific organs and whole body protocols are in some part dependent on the scanner you use, and a complete explanation of the matter is outside the scope of this chapter. Iodine performs as a macro- and micro-vascular enhancer during the first minutes after the i.v. injection, thus allowing the easy recognition of normal and abnormal vascularization patterns of organs and tissues. But minimal dimensions of iodine contrast agent also allow some other kinds of different behavior. The agent is filtered by the kidneys and is excreted with urine in the urinary excretory system some minutes after the injection; also the agent is extracted by the hepatocytes of the liver and excreted with the bile many hours after the injection. A consistent portion of iodine contrast agent leaves the vessels through the spaces between the endothelial cells determining a late interstitial extra vascular enhancement.

Contrast-Enhanced CT in PET-CT (PET-CECT)

The CT part of combined PET-CT imaging is often applied as a whole body low-dose scan without application of i.v. contrast agent (PET-LDCT), which is done primarily for attenuation correction and for anatomic localization of tracer uptake in PET. In some clinical conditions, however, the **contrast enhancement of CT in PET-CT (PET-CECT)** may increase diagnostic accuracy and certainty.

The optimal PET-CECT scanning protocol is still a point of debate. If you plan to use intravenous contrast agents, the injection can be performed in a single-step procedure during the acquisition of whole-body CT data used for attenuation correction or in a two-step approach after completion of the whole body low-dose CT and PET data. The latter approach seems preferable because a multiphase contrast-enhanced CT can be acquired in the region of interest, thus avoiding unnecessary radiation exposure if the PET-LDCT doesn't show any pathologic or doubtful findings, or if it identifies systemic disease.

The benefit of PET-CECT compared to PET-LDCT is more pronounced in those diseases in which surgical intervention or radiation therapy alone are the most commonly used treatments. It has already been shown that combined PET-CECT is the best available diagnostic modality for staging of patients with localized central bronchial tumors. PET imaging warrants a high sensitivity for detection of distant metastasis and CECT allows the exact delineation of mediastinal and chest wall invasion by the primary tumor, as well as the exact demarcation of involved juxtaposed lymph nodes and vessels. Comprehensive information regarding tumor delineation is a precondition for both planning of radiation and surgical treatments, and has a clear benefit, including changes in management as well as in diagnostic confidence.

The results of PET imaging can be optimized if doubtful findings are finally judged on a CECT assessment. This is particularly true if an area of focal increased uptake cannot be attributed only on the basis of low-dose CT to an anatomical structure (for example malignant pancreatic lesion or benign duodenum inflammatory lesion) or if a lesion shows only mild or no increase in FDG uptake. In these cases, a CECT on the region of interest allows lesion detection and characterization.

A full-dose contrast-enhanced CT should also be performed if small lesions in the liver or spleen are suspected by US and no pathologic finding is identified by PET-LDCT. The lack of sensitivity in the detection of such small lesions by PET-LDCT could be due to its lower resolution compared to full-dose CECT.

It should also be emphasized that a fully diagnostic PET-CECT examination results in increased patient radiation exposure as compared to a PET-LDCT examination using only LDCT for attenuation correction of the emission data. Therefore, patient referral for PET-CECT studies should be justified in each case to avoid repeated exposure or overexposure of patients. A PET-CECT scanning should be avoided in patients primarily under consideration for systemic therapy, in patients with recently performed state-of-the-art whole-body CT and in patients referred for therapy monitoring. Finally, if you plan to use intravenous contrast you need to remember that the physician needs to be on site for monitoring and dealing with potential allergic reactions/extravasations. It is necessary to be aware of i.v. contrast contraindications: poor renal function, myeloma, diabetes and others: in these instances it is mandatory to pre-assess the renal function, and take into account alternative approaches.

In cases of diagnostic examination in patients with pelvic or abdominal cancers or in patients with suspected peritoneal metastasis, the use of **oral contrast** is strongly suggested, if not mandatory. Oral contrast allows one to better delineate gastrointestinal organs from surrounding structures, thus improving diagnostic accuracy and confidence. If the administration of oral contrast is planned, the patient should be requested to arrive earlier: contrast drinking starts 90 mins before scanning, 1 cup every 25 minutes, and it is advisable to monitor the drinking schedule. To obtain optimal contrast of the stomach, a last cup of contrast solution is taken just before patient positioning on the table.

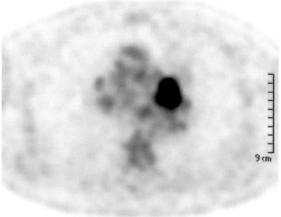

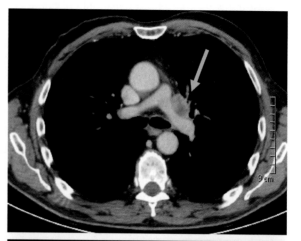

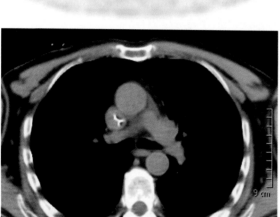

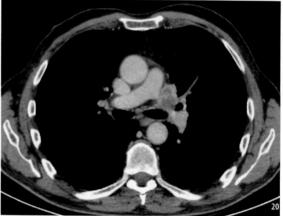

■ PET-CECT images show primary lung cancer and the infiltration of pulmonary artery and bronchial wall

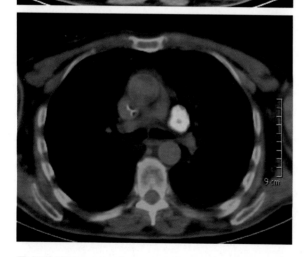

■ PET-CT images show primary lung cancer

Teaching point

PET-CECT may help to assess vessel and bronchial wall invasion. Additional information regarding tumor delineation allows the best surgical approach.

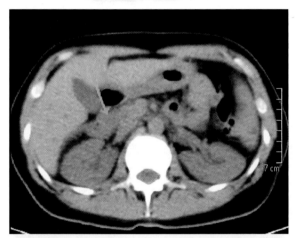

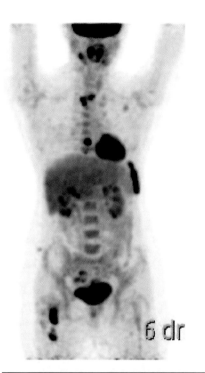

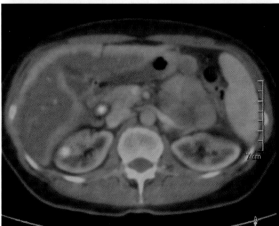

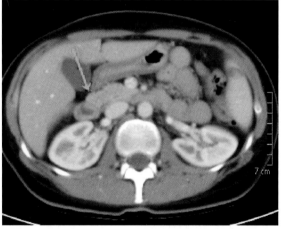

☐ PET-CECT identifies pathologic area in the pancreas

☐ PET-CT shows multiple bone lesions but the images do not allow exact localization of hypermetabolic area in the abdomen

Teaching point

Additional diagnostic contrast enhanced full-dose CT is mandatory in doubtful findings for exact localization of hypermetabolic findings.

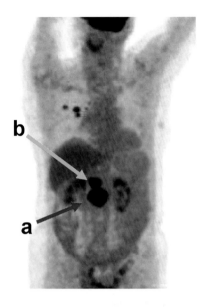

◄ PET-CT images show multiple lung metastasis
and lymph node secondary lesion in the abdomen

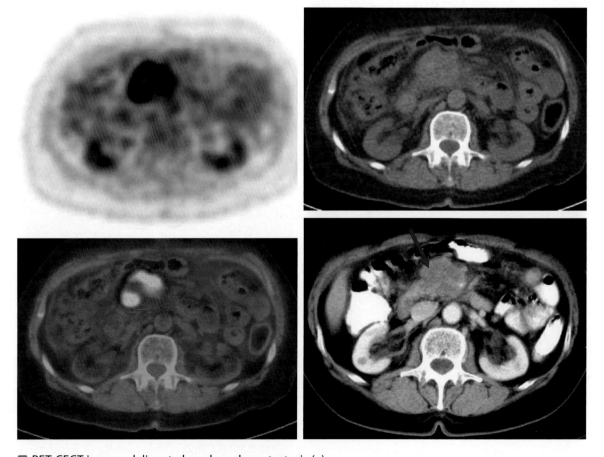

▢ PET-CECT images delineate lymph node metastasis (a)

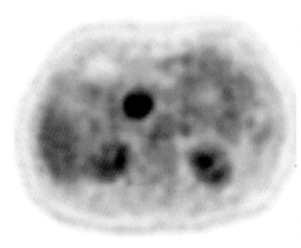
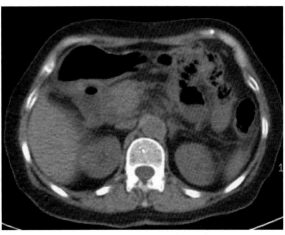

■ PET-CT images identify another hypermetabolic lesion in the abdomen (b)

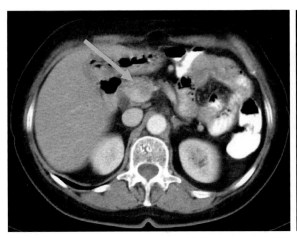
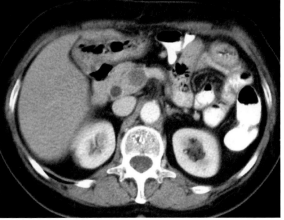

■ CECT images show thrombosis of mesenteric-portal vein confluence

Teaching point

Thrombosis may show FDG uptake. PET-CECT reduces false positive results by better identification of vessels.

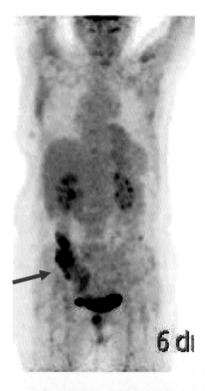

◀ PET-CT images show pathologic uptake in the abdomen suspected for tumor relapse, but also attributable to aspecific bowel uptake

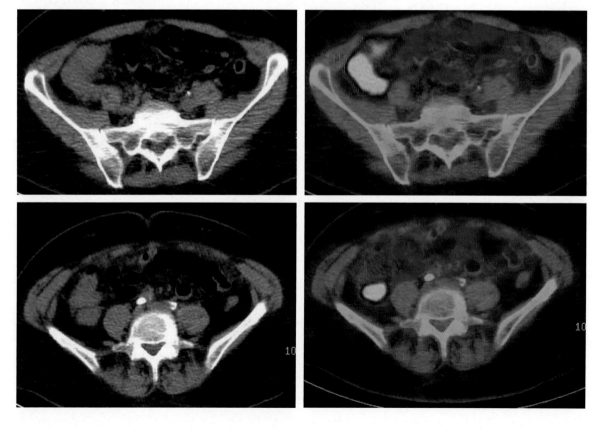

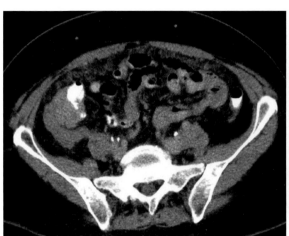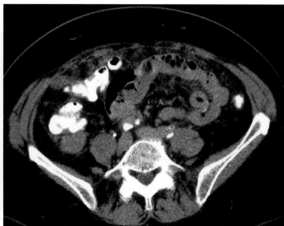

▣ Oral contrasted CT image clearly shows soft tissue implants

Teaching point

Oral contrast allows one to better delineate gastrointestinal organs from surrounding structures, thus improving diagnostic accuracy and confidence. Using oral contrast is mandatory in patients with pelvic or abdominal cancers or in patients with suspected peritoneal metastasis.

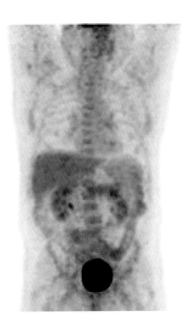

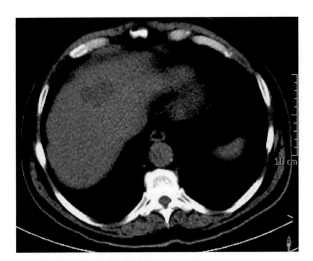

◘ PET findings

area of faint increased uptake in
the liver suspected for residual
disease

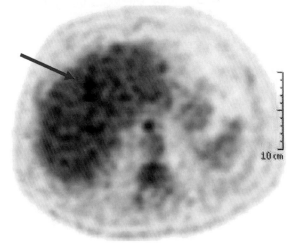

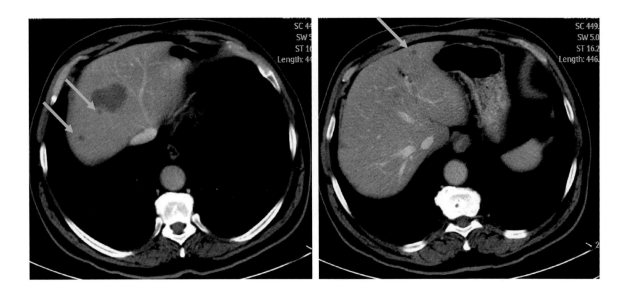

◘ CECT findings

identification of new liver lesions (→ progressive disease)

Teaching point

Diagnosis of small lesions in the liver can be difficult with PET-CT alone. PET-CECT may help to detect small lesions in the liver, spleen or lung.

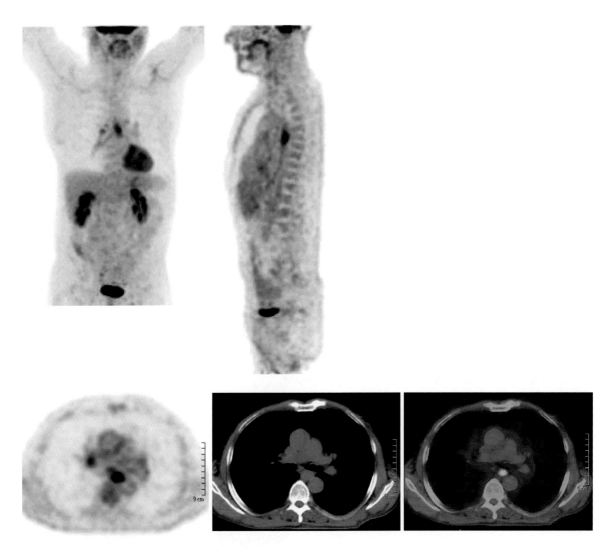

⬛ Intense FDG uptake of primary esophageal cancer shown by PET-CT

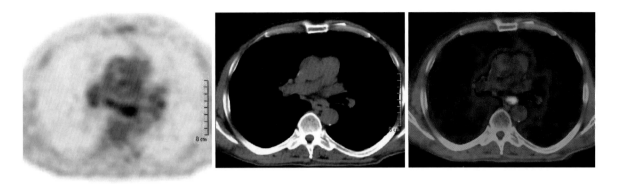

▣ PET-CECT allows the localization of juxtaposed secondary lymph node not identified by low dose CT

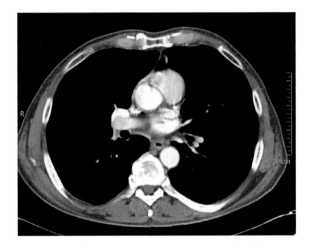

Teaching point

PET-CECT raises diagnostic confidence of PET-CT because of more accurate lesion characterization by exact delineation of the involved lymph nodes.

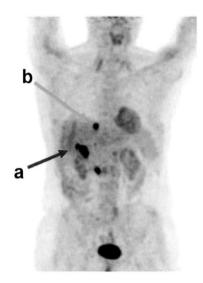

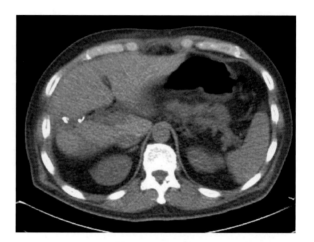

■ PET-CT identifies pathologic hypermetabolic lesion at abdomen

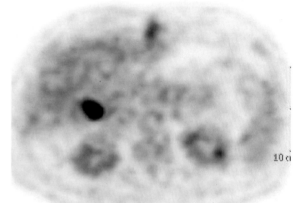

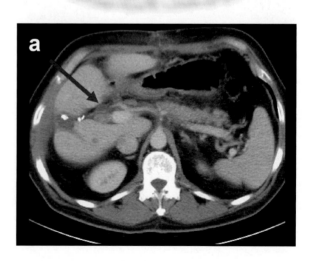

■ PET-CECT identifies pathologic lymph node (a) at the hepatic hilum

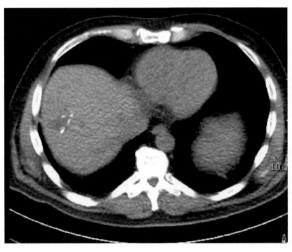
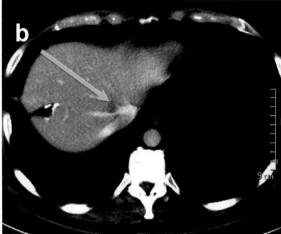
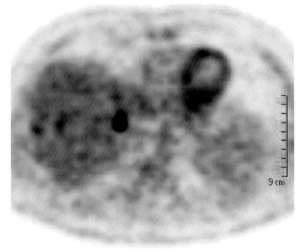

■ PET-CECT delineates the liver lesion (b) from the adjacent vessels

Chapter 3 Pitfalls in FDG PET-CT

Pitfalls in FDG PET-CT

Since FDG-PET is rapidly gaining a crucial role in therapeutic decision-making and management of cancer patients, it is important to clarify the incidence and causes of potential pitfalls.

The most important issue to remember is that ^{18}F-FDG is not a tumor-specific tracer since inflammatory conditions and some benign processes may cause areas of increased FDG uptake. Several examples of potentially misleading inflammatory processes causing false positive results are reported in the literature. Most common sources of such misinterpretations include non-specific inflammation, abscess, sarcoidosis and other granulomatous diseases, post-radiation inflammatory processes, gastritis and colitis. Although the degree of inflammatory process uptake is usually less than the uptake within the neoplastic tissues, there is clearly an overlap between the two conditions and, in some cases, the uptake could even exceed the neoplastic uptake.

Many other benign processes, including uterine fibroids, bladder diverticulum, thymic hyperplasia, atherosclerotic plaque, laryngeal nerve palsy, occult bone infarction, fibrous dysplasia of the bone, adenomatous polyps in the colon and autoimmune diseases such as Grave's disease or physiological conditions like muscle contraction, brown adipose tissue and even the ovulation and the normal menstrual cycle may cause increased FDG uptake.

Physiologic radiotracer activity in bowel loops, the urinary system, blood vessels, pelvic kidney and bone marrow can similarly lead to false-positive interpretations.

However, many of these above-described causes of misinterpretation can be properly recognized. Proper patient preparation and scanning protocol are needed for accurate PET-CT imaging. Four to six hours fasting time prior to PET scanning is necessary, and oral hydration is recommended. Muscle stress, tension and movement during the uptake portion should be minimized to decrease muscle uptake. It is also important to reduce FDG accumulation within the urinary bladder if pelvic malignancies are studied. Patients should void completely immediately prior to the start of scanning and by imaging the pelvis early in the study. Metallic objects (keys and wallets, etc.) of the patients should be removed and patient movements during the PET scanning should be avoided.

Some potential causes of false positive results like bowel or tonsil uptake, or activity of blood vessels, can be easily interpreted only by recognizing the normal FDG uptake distribution: in these cases the experience of the PET reader is clearly crucial.

Many of the pitfalls that have plagued FDG PET imaging, like correct identification of brown fat or interpretation of focal bone uptake due to non-malignant processes can be avoided by using PET-CT systems. The new PET-CT scanners allow one to localize anatomically areas of increased FDG uptake, thus improving diagnostic accuracy and confidence of functional PET imaging. PET-CT scanners are also extremely useful for interpretation of areas of FDG uptake in the bowel.

Finally, relevant history and data collected before PET scanning may help to avoid many causes of false positive results like recent fracture, phase of ovulation or menstrual cycle, recent surgery or radiation therapy, presence of benign thyroid or lung disease or any other nonneoplastic pathologic condition (for example acute or chronic infection). The interpretation of PET scans is improved when relevant studies and clinical data are considered and other diagnostic radiologic investigations are reviewed.

Abdomen

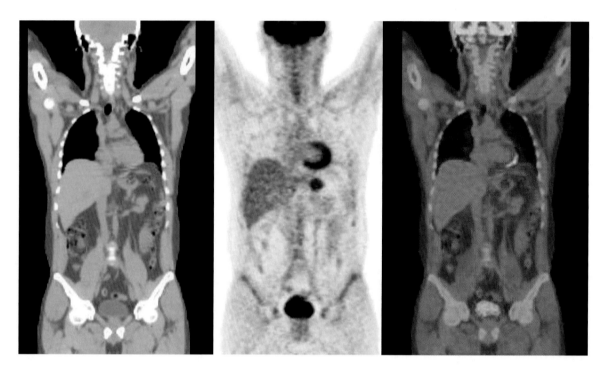

◘ FDG uptake in gastric region. Diagnosis: gastritis

Teaching point

FDG is taken up by inflammatory processes, and due to the high frequency of gastritis in oncological patients, an increased FDG uptake at stomach can frequently be seen.

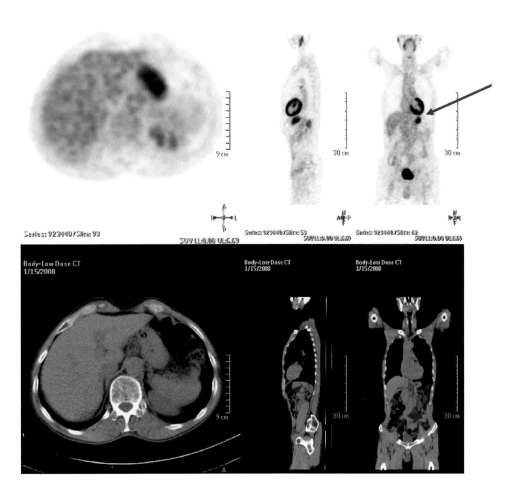

■ Intense FDG uptake in the stomach. Diagnosis: gastritis

Teaching point

FDG uptake is likely to be intense in the presence of clinically evident gastritis. In inflammatory diseases the uptake is usually diffuse to the entire stomach: in cases of focal uptake, further investigations can be recommended.

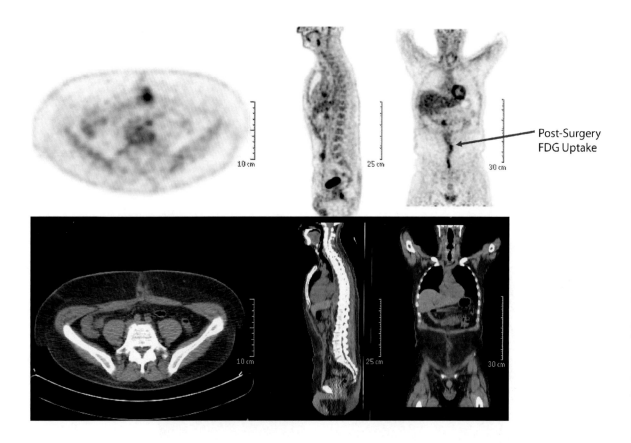

Post-Surgery
FDG Uptake

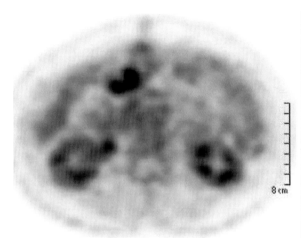

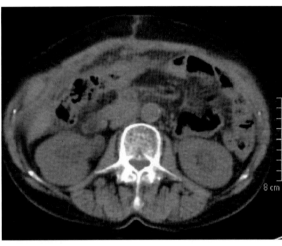

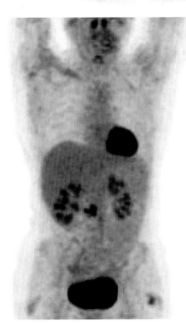

◘ FDG uptake due to inflammatory changes due to recent termino-terminal anastomosis of bowel

Teaching point

Surgery will affect FDG uptake due to inflammatory processes. Increased uptake is almost constant for several months at scar level, but also near the surgical bed. It may therefore be difficult to identify the local recurrence of disease within a few months of intervention.

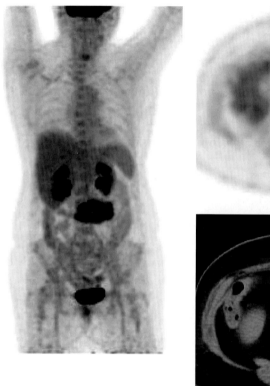
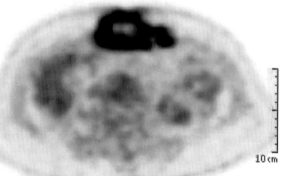
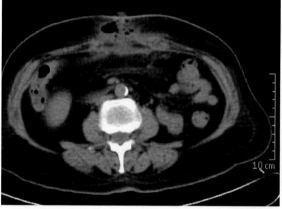

◘ FDG uptake due to abscess

Teaching point

The presence of a clinically evident inflammatory process will always determine an increased uptake of FDG. Therefore, PET cannot be used to characterize an uncertain CT finding at the same level of an abscess, but nevertheless can be used to evaluate the rest of the body.

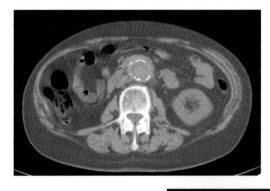 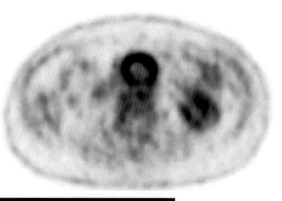

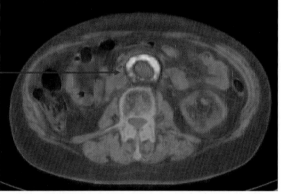

Intense FDG Uptake Due
To Aortic Aneurysm

Teaching point

FDG is probably taken up by inflammatory
cells of atheromasic plaque that infiltrated
the arterial walls and the soft tissue mass.
This case indicates that FDG-PET is a useful
method for localization of inflammatory
lesion in patients with unspecific clinical
findings and laboratory data. Other works
suggest a possible correlation between
FDG uptake by the aneurysm wall and the
triggering of processes leading to rupture.

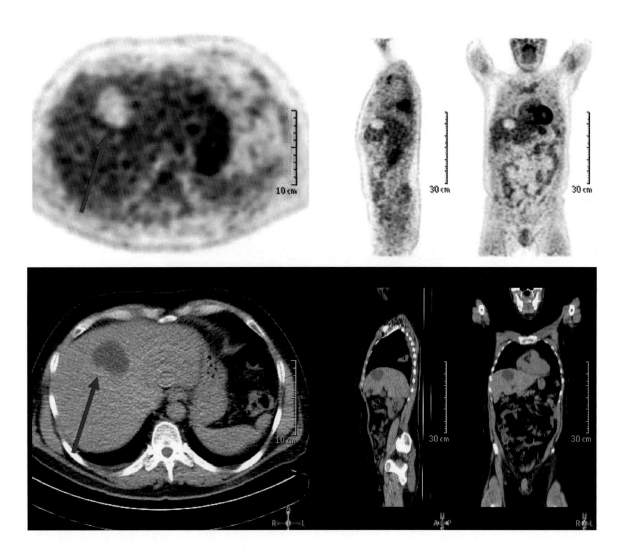

Teaching point

Cystic lesions appear as cold areas at PET, as cysts do not show any uptake of FDG.

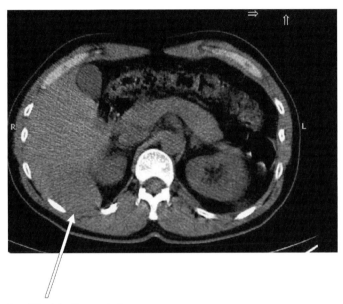

Focal Nodular Hyperplasia

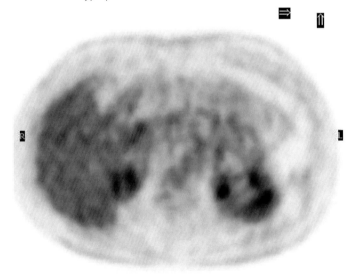

Teaching point

Other liver lesions (such as focal nodular hyperplasia) do not show any increased uptake of FDG, and therefore will not be detectable on FDG PET.

Bone

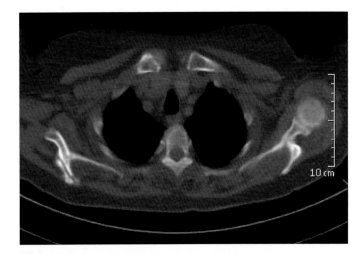

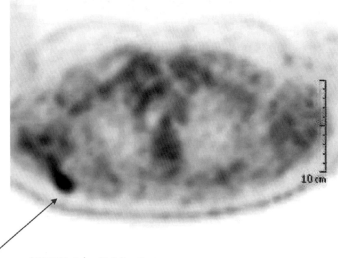

Increased FDG Uptake At A Fracture

Teaching point

Whole-body FDG PET is an important tool for the imaging of cancer, including skeletal metastases. False-positive results can occur in benign diseases such as fractures, especially in recent lesion or in non-consolidated lesion.

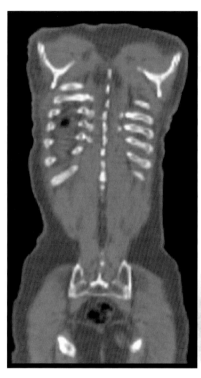
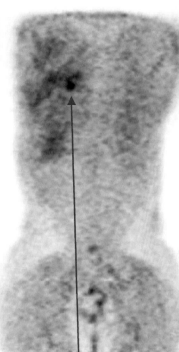
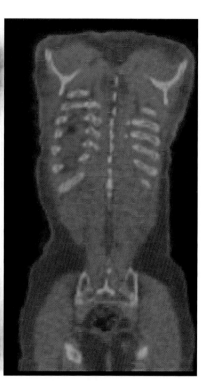

Increased FDG Uptake
At A Fracture

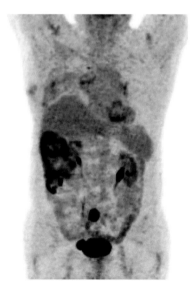

Teaching point

Fracture can occur with relatively high frequency after surgical approaches, as in this case. In this particula patient a number of potential pitfalls can be observed (scar uptake, non-specific bilateral hilar uptake and fracture focal uptake.

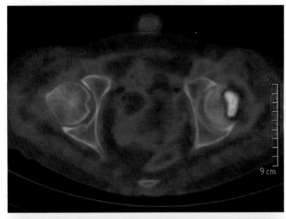

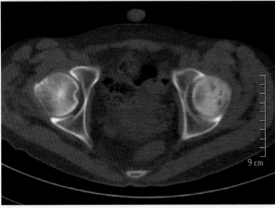

◼ Increased FDG uptake due to osteonecrosis of the femoral head

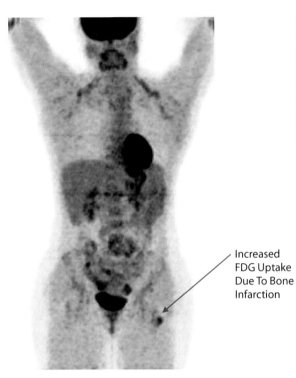

Increased
FDG Uptake
Due To Bone
Infarction

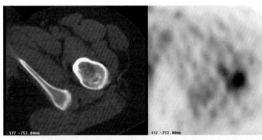

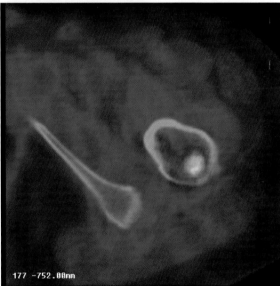

Teaching point

The lesion was not a metastasis even if
it cannot be distinguished by the PET
semeiotic. There is only one case report
in the literature: "bone infarct can take up
FDG, probably as a result of an inflammatory
process".

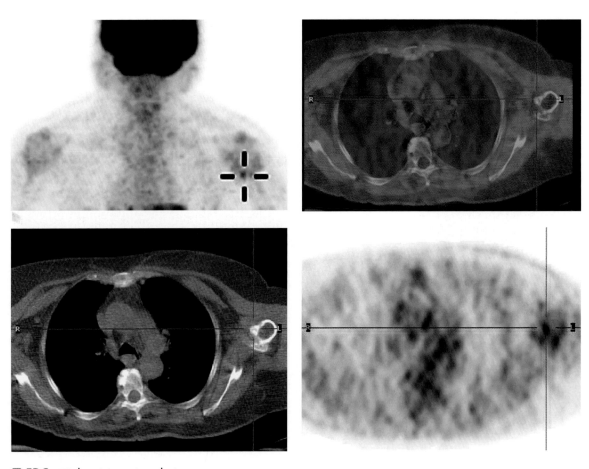

■ FDG uptake at an osteophyte

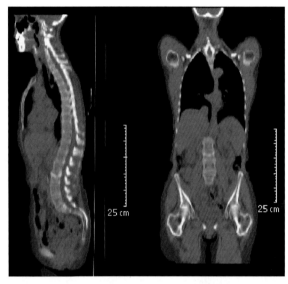

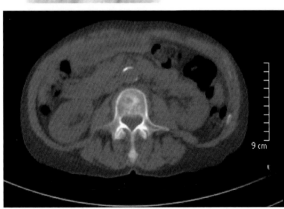

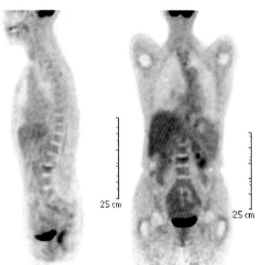

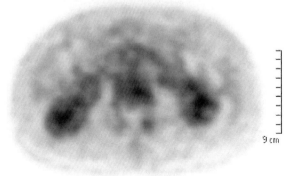

◘ FDG uptake due to the degenerative changes of the spine

Teaching point

FDG increased uptake can be observed in degenerative spine disease.

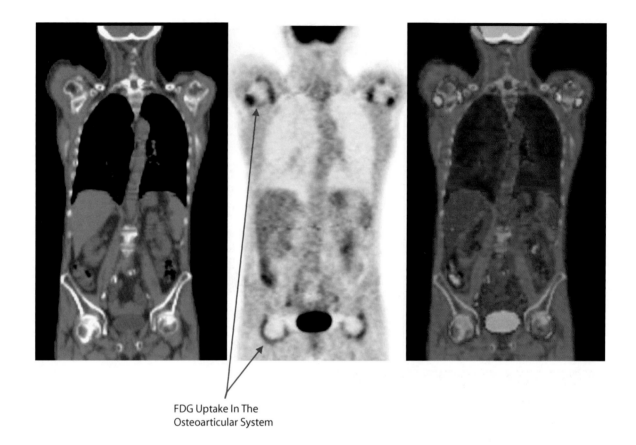

FDG Uptake In The
Osteoarticular System

Teaching point

FDG increased uptake can be observed
in all pathological situations causing a joint
inflammation.

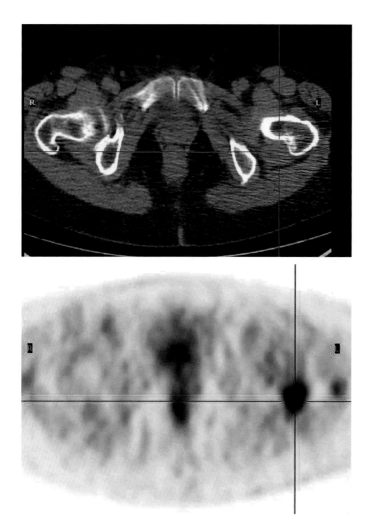

◨ Intense FDG uptake due to bursitis

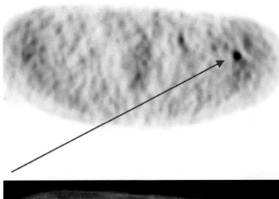

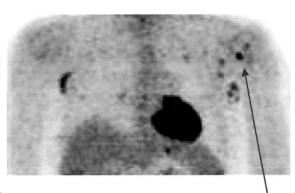

Intense FDG Uptake At Articulary Level

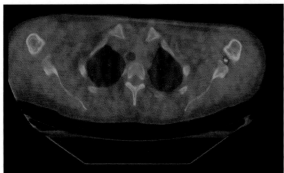

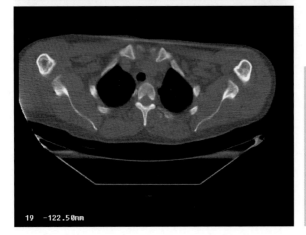

19 -122.50mm

Teaching point

The introduction of PET-CT systems enables both morphological and metabolic imaging to be performed in a single session, reducing false positive findings and inconclusive studies, thus increasing diagnostic accuracy.

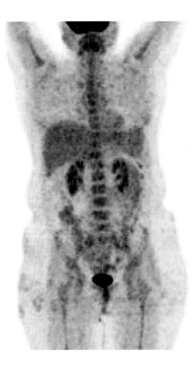

◘ Diffuse bone marrow FDG uptake in a patient with lymphoma undergoing treatment

Teaching point

Increased FDG uptake at bone marrow can frequently be observed as a consequence of chemotherapy, or other therapy (CSF) or various conditions (anemia).

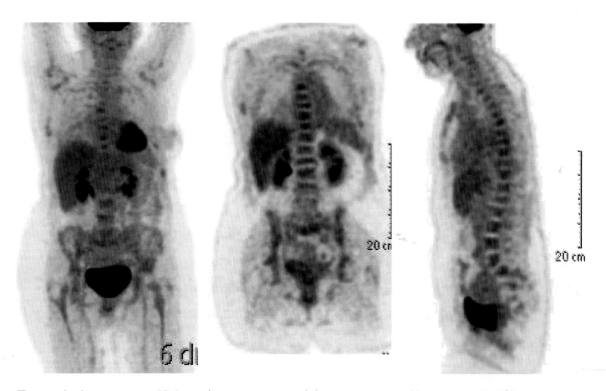

◘ Irregular bone marrow FDG uptake in a patient with breast cancer and bone marrow infiltration

Teaching point

Less frequently increased FDG uptake at bone marrow may be related to cancer infiltration, but even in diffuse infiltration some dishomogeneous uptake can be seen.

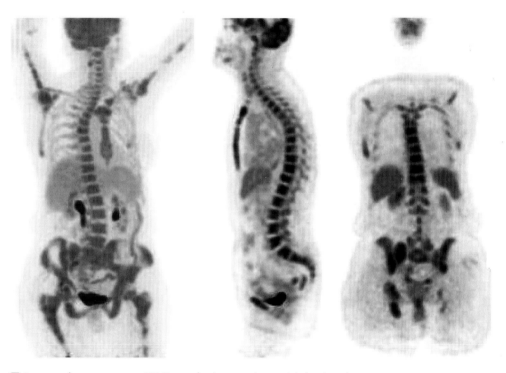

◘ Intense bone marrow FDG uptake in a patient with leukemia

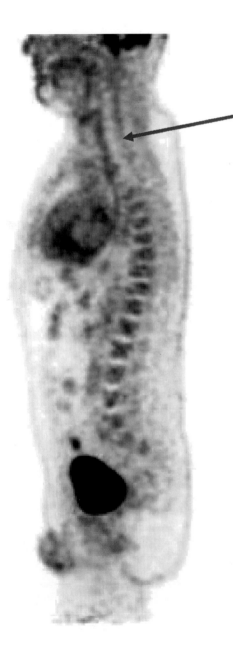

Reduced Bone Marrow FDG
Uptake In A Patient With
Lymphoma Treated With
External Radiation Treatment

Teaching point

Reduced FDG uptake at bone marrow can
frequently be observed as a consequence of
radiation therapy.

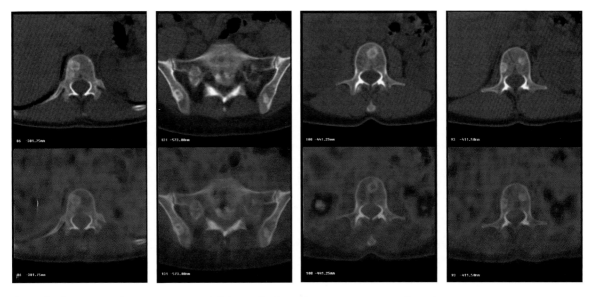

■ Lack of FDG uptake in a patient with bone lesions due to metastases from breast cancer

Teaching point

In few case of advanced stage cancer or other cause of severe compromising of general status, bone lesions can be missed at PET.

Head and Neck

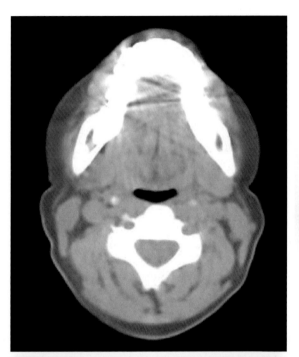

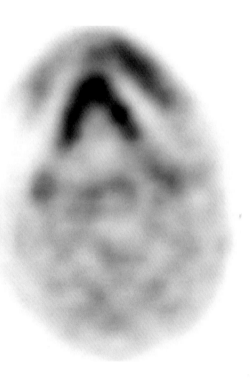

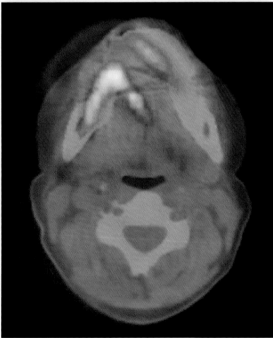

⬛ Artifact due to movement: wrong fusion between PET and CT images

Teaching point

Each patient movement during the exam execution, in particular between CT and PET scans, implies a movement artifact. This mistaken alignment could set errors in the morphological localization of hypermetabolic areas, especially in regions characterized by unique complexity, such as the head and neck. Head restraints minimizing movement is one option, but other alternative strategies have been developed.

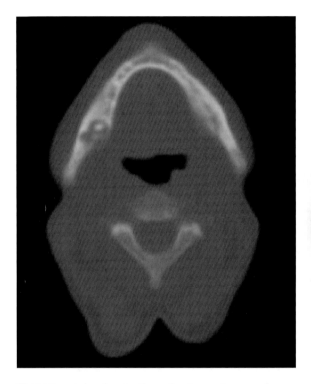

▣ FDG uptake due to the odontogenic granuloma

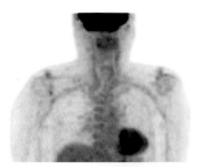

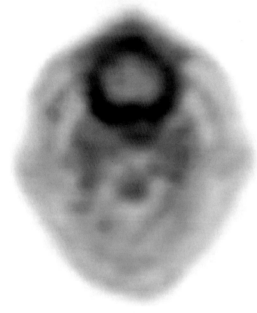

◨ FDG uptake due to mucositis

Teaching point

This scan was carried out a few weeks after external radiation therapy, which is a well known cause of inflammatory changes.

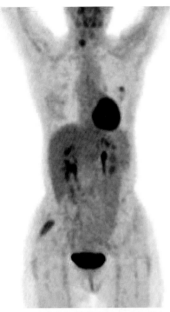

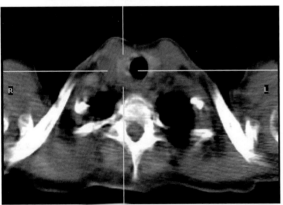

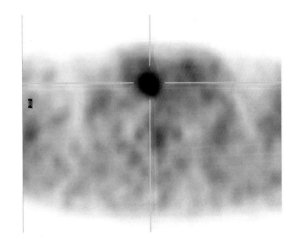

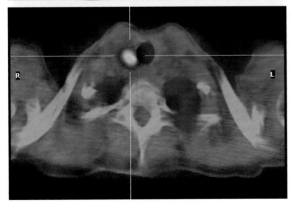

73

Teaching point

Benign thyroid disease may show intense FDG uptake.

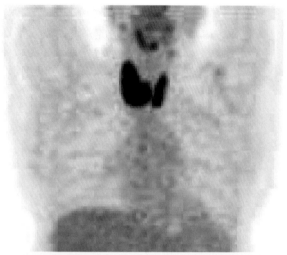

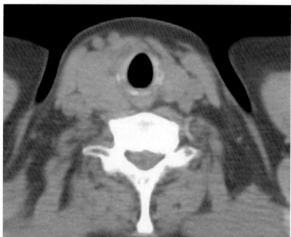

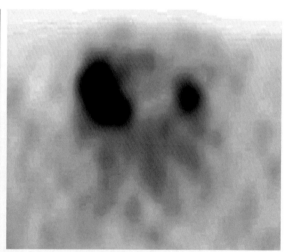

■ Intense FDG uptake in multinodular goiter

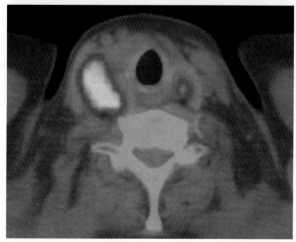

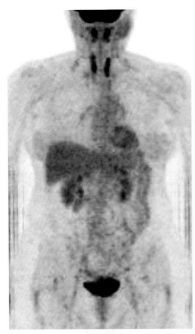

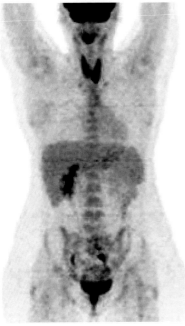

Teaching point

Inflammatory lesions are well known causes of increased FDG uptake; a frequent site of unknown chronic inflammation is the thyroid gland.

🔲 Increased FDG uptake in thyroiditis

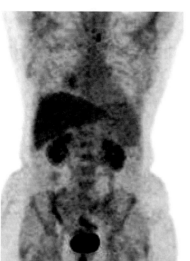

Teaching point

Occult thyroid cancer is an occasional incidental finding during imaging exams or surgery for other indications. Despite most nodules being benign, in the presence of focal suspect findings further investigations are mandatory (this case turned out to be a malignant cancer at FNA).

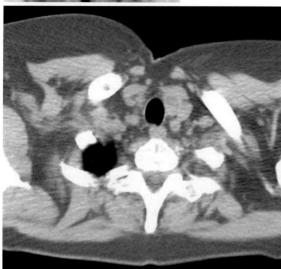

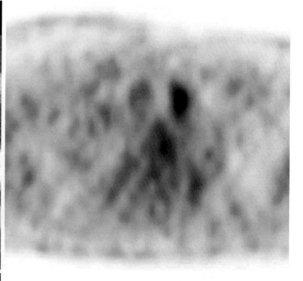

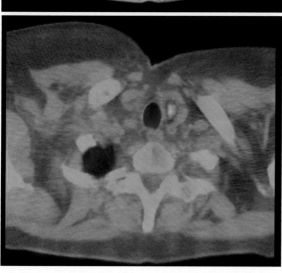

◻ Focal FDG uptake in the thyroid nodule

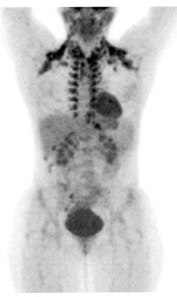

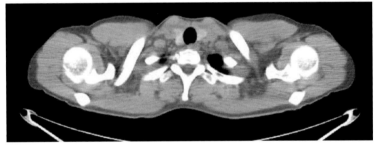

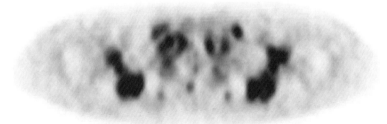

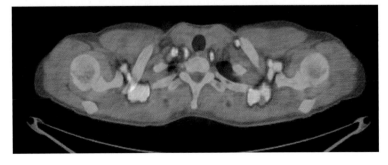

◘ FDG Uptake in brown fat

Chest

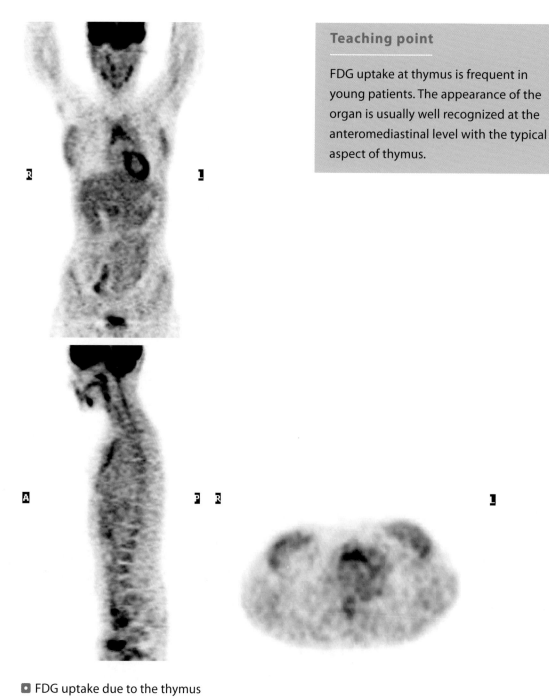

Teaching point

FDG uptake at thymus is frequent in young patients. The appearance of the organ is usually well recognized at the anteromediastinal level with the typical aspect of thymus.

◼ FDG uptake due to the thymus

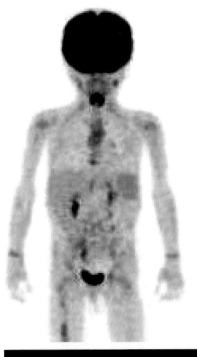

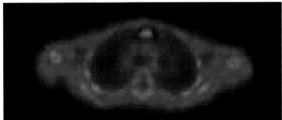

◘ FDG uptake due to the thymus

Teaching point

FDG uptake at thymus is particularly evident in the pediatric population.

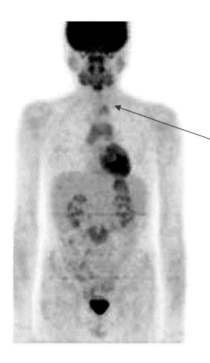

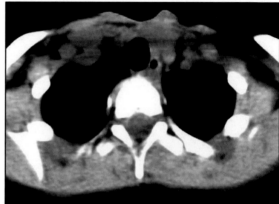

FDG Uptake Due To The Ectopic Left Lobe Of Thymus

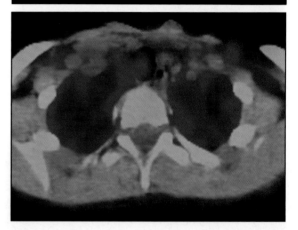

Teaching point

FDG uptake at thymus may be challenging to recognize in anatomic variants.

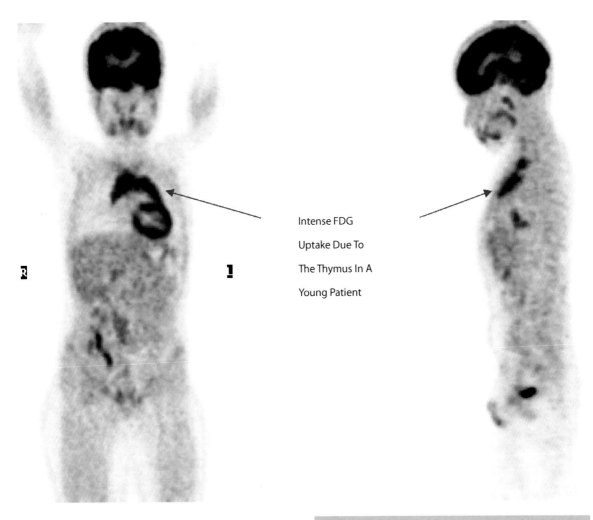

Intense FDG

Uptake Due To

The Thymus In A

Young Patient

Teaching point

FDG uptake at thymus can be very intense
in cases of young lymphoma patients
after treatment due to thymic reactive
hyperplasia.

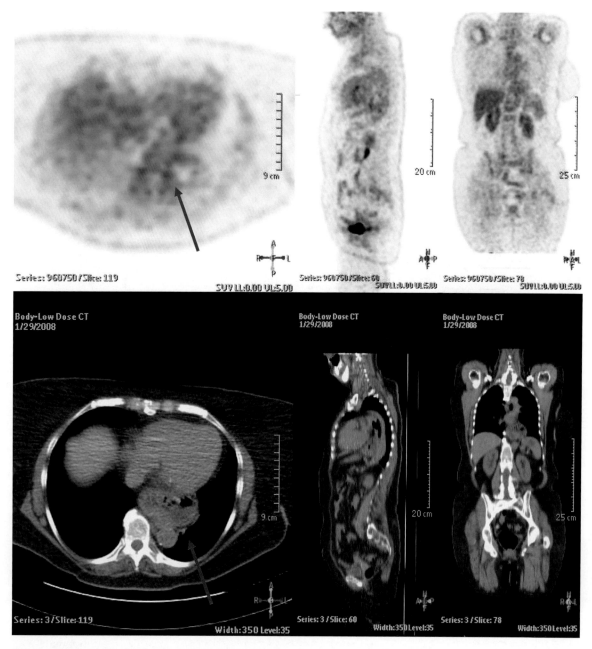

Series: 960750/Slice: 119

SUV LL:0.00 UL:5.00

Series: 960750/Slice: 60

SUV LL:0.00 UL:5.00

Series: 960750/Slice: 78

SUV LL:0.00 UL:5.00

Body-Low Dose CT
1/29/2008

Body-Low Dose CT
1/29/2008

Body-Low Dose CT
1/29/2008

Series: 3/Slice: 119

Width: 350 Level: 35

Series: 3/Slice: 60

Width: 350 Level: 35

Series: 3/Slice: 78

Width: 350 Level: 35

▣ Mild FDG uptake due to the gastric hiatal hernia

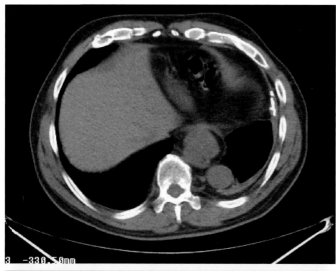

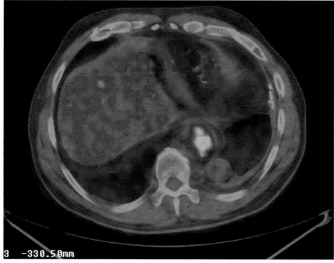

◘ Intense FDG uptake due to hiatal hernia

Teaching point

Inflammatory lesions are well known causes of increased FDG uptake; in many cases a careful evaluation of patient history, and attention to CT images, can help avoid false positive report.

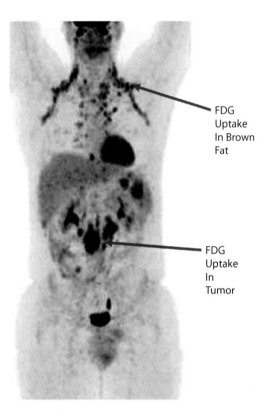

FDG
Uptake
In Brown
Fat

FDG
Uptake
In
Tumor

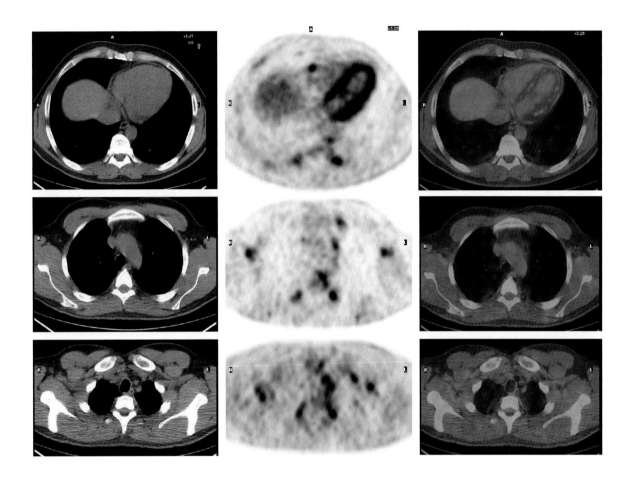

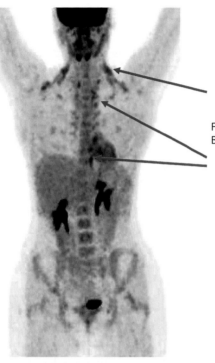

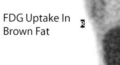

FDG Uptake In Brown Fat

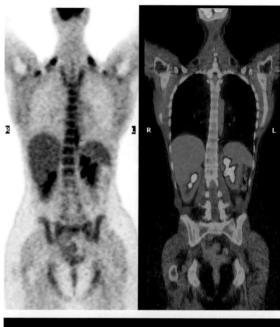

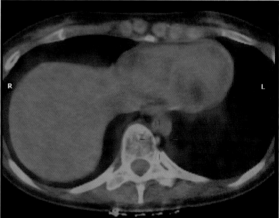

Teaching point

Degree of FDG uptake at brown fat can be variable, and sometimes not easy to identify in unusual locations. PET-CT is extremely useful in locating the uptake in areas of fat density.

FDG Uptake
Due To
Esophagitis

10 c

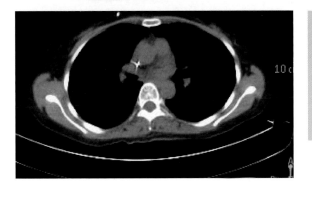

10 c

Teaching point

Increased uptake of FDG can be observed
in the presence of inflammatory disease of
the esophagus; it is usually diffuse and of
moderate degree.

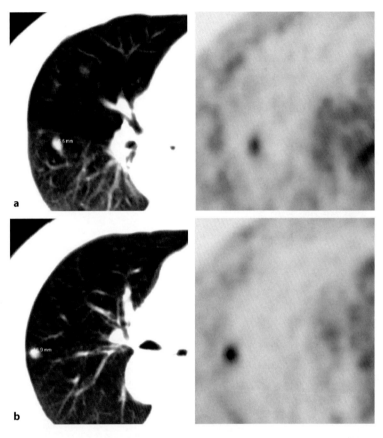

◘ Different degree of FDG uptake in lung metastases

Teaching point

Partial volume effect may strongly influence the uptake of small lesions. Particular care has to be paid when evaluating lesions < 8 mm at the limit of PET resolution. The degree of uptake is different (a SUV max = 3; b SUV max = 6) despite similar dimension and same histology.

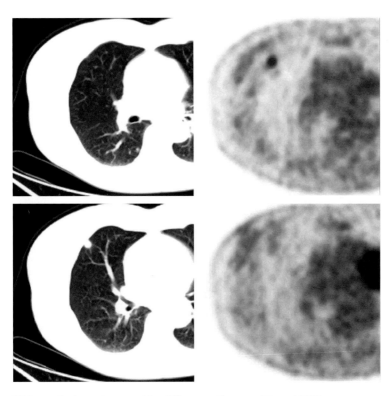

◘ Lung lesion observed in different slices at CT and PET

Teaching point

Respiratory movement occurs during the exam execution, thus exact correspondence of PET and CT findings cannot be absolute, especially at lung bases. In any case, however, a lung nodule can be observed with PET and missed with CT, due to the better spatial resolution of CT.

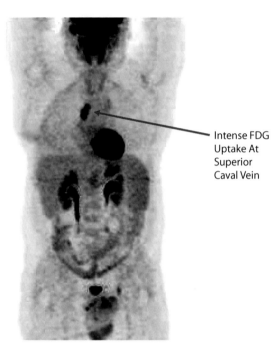

Intense FDG
Uptake At
Superior
Caval Vein

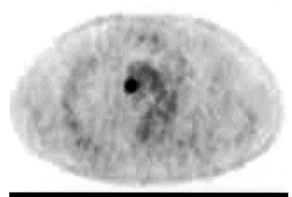

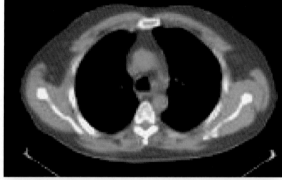

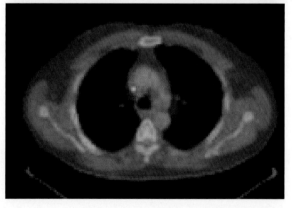

Teaching point

Although FDG-PET is widely used in
differentiating between malignant and
benign diseases, it has to be remembered
that benign entities can demonstrate
high accumulations of FDG. In this case
the intense uptake was due to a recent
thrombus.

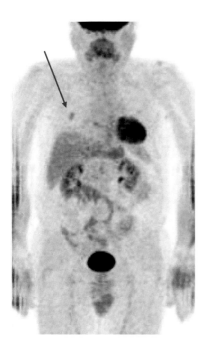

◘ Mild FDG uptake at a rib due to recent fracture

Teaching point

During the anamnesis it is fundamental to ask the patient if he/she had any fractures, crashes or falls in the past several months.

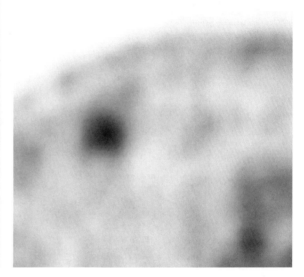

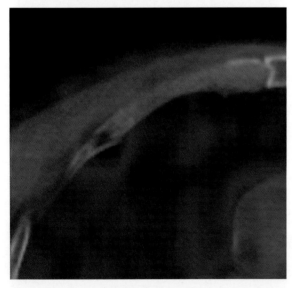

◼ Mild FDG uptake at a rib due to recent fracture

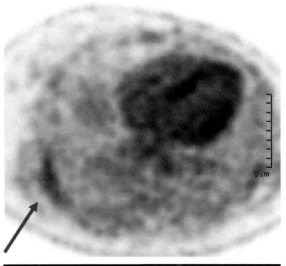

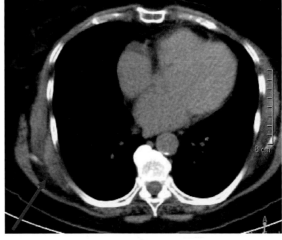

◘ Faint FDG muscle uptake due fibroelastoma dorsi

Teaching point

Some benign soft tissue processes may show increased FDG uptake; PET-CT is very useful in identifying anatomic abnormalities and characterizing some benign lesions.

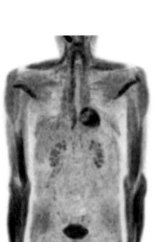

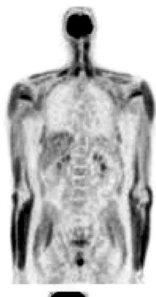
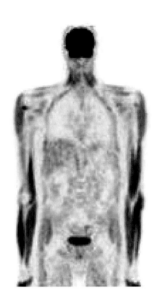
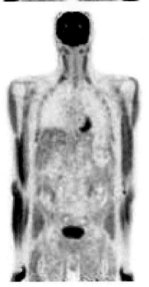
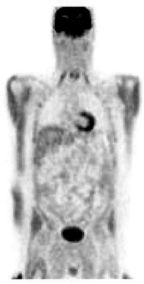

■ FDG uptake in muscles due to food intake prior to scanning

Teaching point

Food intake prior to PET scanning may cause increased glucose uptake in muscle or other soft tissue and compromise the sensitivity of the scan. If the blood glucose levels are high (> 200 ng/ml) and cannot be lowered on the day of the study, a patient may have to be rescheduled.

Pelvis

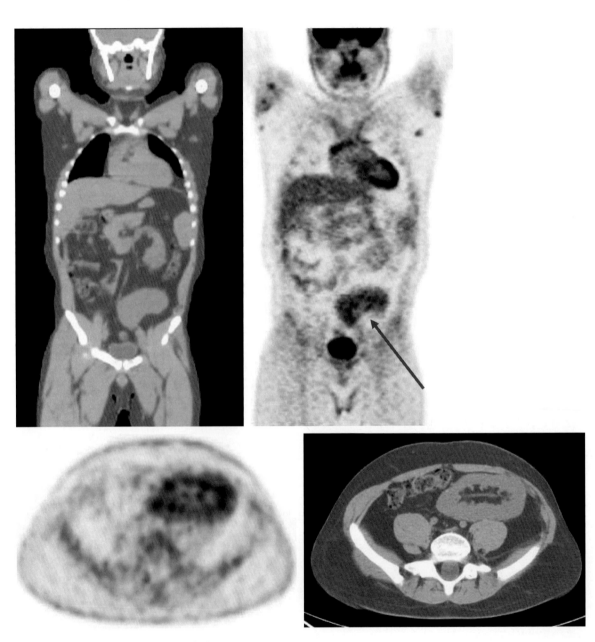

□ FDG uptake in a transplanted kidney

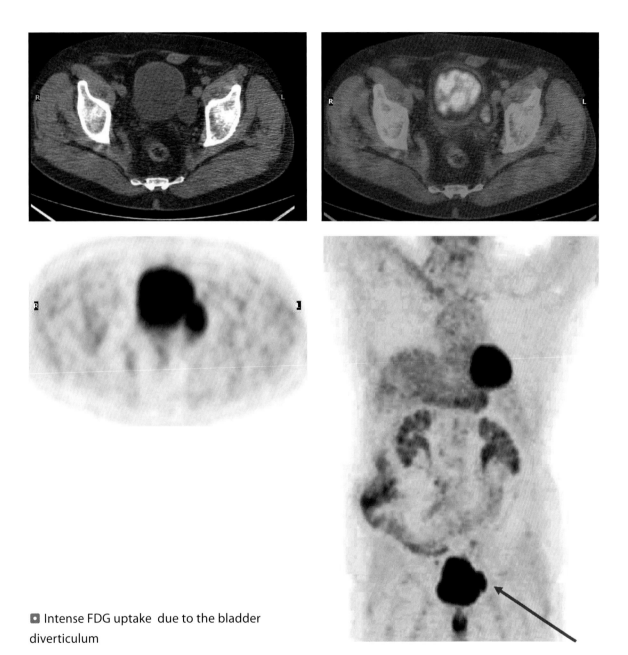

◘ Intense FDG uptake due to the bladder diverticulum

▣ FDG uptake in the bowel

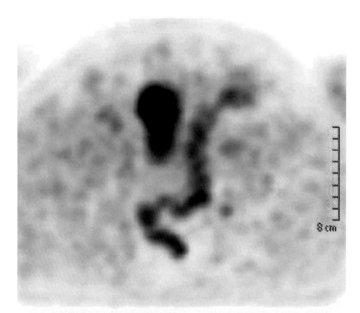

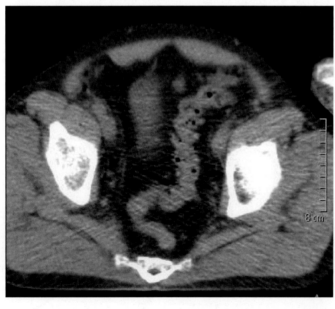

Teaching point

Diverticulosis or more commonly diverticulitis may cause FDG uptake.

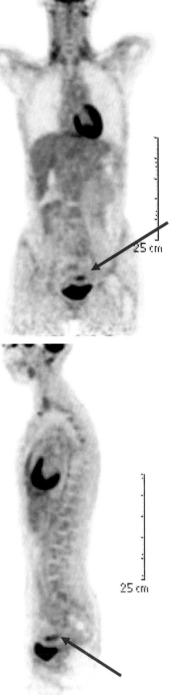

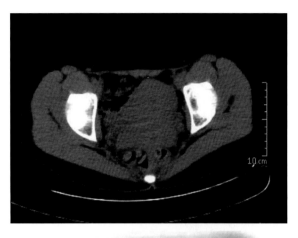

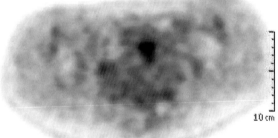

Teaching point

Menstruation can determine focal FDG uptake. Pelvic increased FDG uptake can be observed in the endometrium (menstrual phase) and ovary (ovulation); also uptakes can be observed in premenopausal women and in cases of intrauterine abnormal bleeding (e.g. benign tumors).

◘ FDG uptake in the uterus

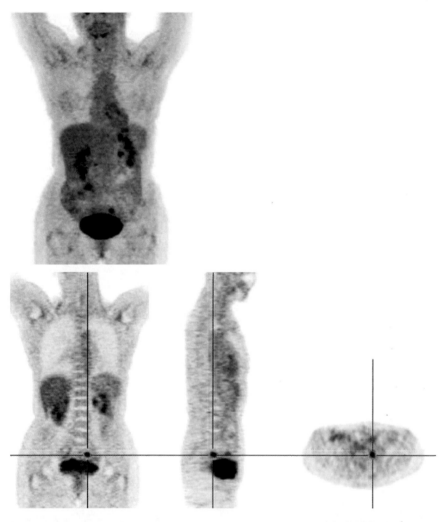

◘ FDG focal uptake in the pelvis

Teaching point

The focal increased FDG uptake was considered suspect for neoplastic lesion, and due to its unusual site a biopsy was performed. The lesion turned out to be a benign uterine leiomyoma.

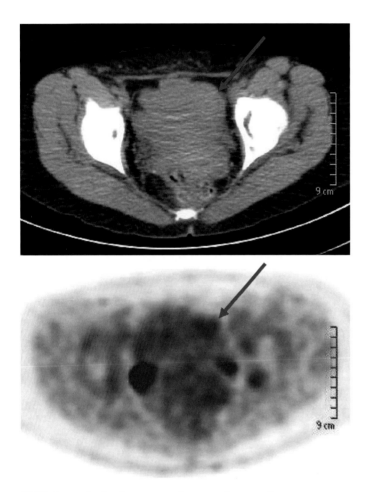

◘ FDG uptake in the uterus due to miomatosis

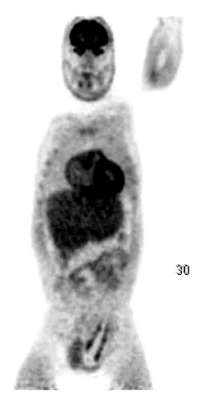

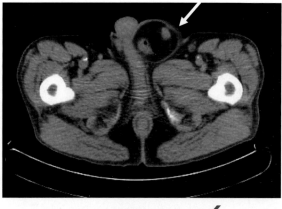

30

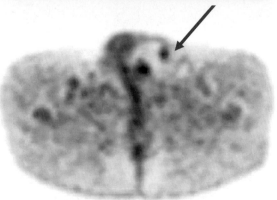

◙ FDG uptake in the pelvis due to inguinal hernia

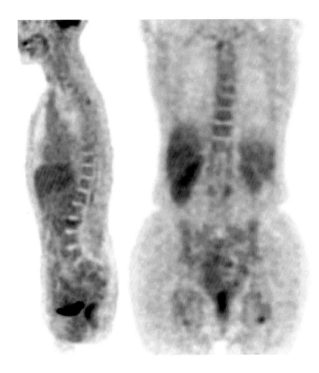

◧ Pelvis FDG uptake in the rectum

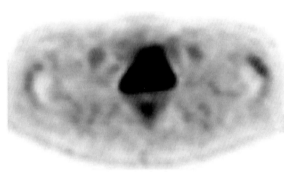

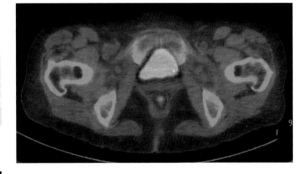

Teaching point

The rectum may show physiological intense FDG uptake, not necessarily related to malignancy.

Chapter 4   PET-CT in Oncology

PET-CT in Oncology

FDG PET allows one to study in vivo tissue metabolism, and thus to demonstrate malignant tumors as hypermetabolic lesions, showing an increase of tracer uptake. At present 18F radiolabelled fluorodeoxyglucose (FDG) is the most employed compound in the clinical practice.

Cancer cells are known to have increased anaerobic glycolytic activity and higher expression of glucose transporters. Many papers have demonstrated a relevant impact of FDG PET on staging of many neoplastic diseases, and a better accuracy of FDG PET in comparison with conventional diagnostic methods for therapy response evaluation and for relapse identification in many cancers.

PET images, however, provide limited anatomical data, and this represents a significant drawback, as exact localization of lesions may be difficult in many cases on the basis of PET images alone. Therefore, the introduction of PET-CT hybrid systems, allowing one to obtain both morphological and metabolic imaging in a single session, reduced the incidence of false positive findings and inconclusive studies, thus increasing diagnostic accuracy.

Currently, PET-CT imaging is employed in several oncologic diseases, namely non small cell lung cancer, colo-rectal cancer, malignant lymphoma, melanoma, head and neck cancer, oesophageal cancer, cervical cancer, unknown primary cancer, breast cancer, ovarian cancer, thyroid cancer, bone tumors, seminoma, pancreatic cancer, gastric cancer and many others. Many American and European reports describe FDG PET appropriate indications for each neoplastic disease, in the different clinical settings.

Diagnosis

At present the use of PET is limited to the characterization of the solitary pulmonary nodule (SPN) and to the identification of cancer of unknown primary (CUP).

Most lung nodules are discovered incidentally on chest radiographs, and 15% to 75% of such nodules are malignant, depending on the population studied.

Conventional imaging, and in particular multislice CT, represents the first step for localizing the lesion within the lung parenchyma, and CT density characteristics sometimes can find occult calcification or spiculation, indicative for benign cause or malignancy, respectively. Otherwise FDG PET is suggested to identify malignant lesions on the basis of glucolytic metabolism. There is a large amount of data in the literature regarding the usefulness of PET for this indication.

Whole-body PET-CT using 18F-FDG has also been successfully used for identifying CUP of the most common histologies, namely adenocarcinomas, squamous cell carcinomas and poorly differentiated carcinomas.

Staging

The indication for the use of PET imaging for staging is definitely supported by the literature for only few tumors, in particular non small cell lung cancer (NSCLC) and in selected cases of head and neck, oesophageal and breast cancer, as well as in some cases of melanoma and lymphoma.

The definition of NSCLC staging often requires invasive procedures and multiple tests. Whole-body positron-emission tomography may simplify and improve the evaluation of patients affected by this tumor. Mediastinoscopy is still the gold standard for mediastinal staging, even if it is an invasive procedure and not all mediastinal lymph nodes can be easily accessed. FDG PET-CT has been shown to be clinically useful in N and M staging: the use of PET modifies the staging of up to 50% of patients and thus has an unquestionably positive effect on treatment.

T staging of esophageal cancer is usually made at endoscopic biopsy, and CT or magnetic resonance imaging (MRI) are used to demonstrate infiltration of adjacent structures, distant adenopathy and metastases, even if PET-CT seems to provide more information for the initial treatment stratification of patients, in particular by identifying distant lymphatic and hematogenous metastases.

Head and neck carcinoma staging is very complex, and this fact is confirmed by the discordance in published literature. Clinical N0 is a critical situation, as detection of metastatic disease will exclude patients from curative surgical therapy. CT and MR provide excellent anatomic detail but poorly identify unenlarged lymph nodes harboring metastatic disease, while FDG-PET may detect a greater number of lesions. Similarly in esophageal cancer PET is useful for the purpose of N and M staging, with a direct impact on patient management.

Also, patients with advanced disease may benefit from staging PET, as in breast cancer. Sentinel node biopsy (SNB) is currently employed in staging axillary lymph nodes in early breast cancer, but in patients with advanced disease PET-CT has a relevant role to accurately evaluate the extent of the disease.

Response to Therapy

Structural changes in tumor volume are used to assess drug action as a surrogate endpoint for other measures of clinical benefit such as disease-free and overall survival. Moreover, in routine practice clinicians are keen to use volume changes to modify the therapeutic approach.

Since tissue metabolism changes occur before morphological modifications, changes in tumor FDG uptake has largely been used to evaluate response to therapy. A typical example is malignant lymphomas, where anatomical imaging after completion of therapy often reveals residual masses that could represent either persistent disease or fibrotic tissue. Identification of residual disease after radio- or chemotherapy is clearly influencing further treatment options. Positive FDG PET findings after therapy completion in patients affected by lymphoma is a strong predictor of relapse, while a negative PET study has been demonstrated to be an excellent predictor of good prognosis. Several studies have considered the utility of FDG-PET for early response evaluation during the treatment. Early identification of chemotherapy resistant lymphoma patients provides a basis for alternative treatment strategies.

Chemotherapy is currently the treatment of choice for patients with metastatic solid tumors, such as breast, colorectal, ovarian, lung cancer and many others, possibly in combination with surgery. It is widely accepted that response assessment by changes in tumor size (using conventional imaging) requires a longer period and is frequently less accurate than changes in metabolism as demonstrated by PET. FDG PET can predict the response as soon as after a few cycles of chemotherapy for metastatic breast cancer, resulting in a valid tool for prognostic stratification. Also, patients affected by NSCLC with stages III and IV are usually treated with chemotherapy or chemoradiotherapy, and again there is the need for therapy response monitoring, but conventional imaging cannot reliably distinguish necrotic tumor or fibrotic scars from residual tumor tissue. Management of locally advanced rectal cancer includes a treatment with chemoradiotherapy before surgery. Several works in the literature underline the importance of FDG PET in assessing neo-adjuvant chemoradiotherapy response due to its intrinsic capacity to identify precocious changes in tumor behavior, and FDG PET has been reported to be superior to CT and MRI in early prediction of pathologic responses to preoperative treatment. This approach of assessment of therapy response with PET can be extended to several other solid tumors, and a growing number of works can be found in the literature. The usefulness of PET in this setting is likely to be increased by the diffusion of targeted therapy. As an example, one of the principal mechanisms of communication between cells is the binding of polypeptide ligands to cell surface receptors possessing tyrosine kinase (TK) activity. Though many actions of these receptors involve physiological processes, perturbation of TK signalling can result in malignant transformation. During the last few decades, these signalling networks have been studied in detail and finally pharmacological agents targeted at key molecules have been produced and have rapidly become part of the standard care for common tumors like breast, colorectal, ovarian, lung, head and neck. Also, multi-target agents have been introduced and have yielded promising results, and new agents are being developed. Until now, no predictor of response to target therapy has been validated, yet the selection of patients who are likely to benefit from TK inhibitors is mandatory not only for clinical but also for economic reasons, and molecular imaging with PET could be proposed as tools for this purpose.

Relapse

Routine oncologic follow-up includes clinical evaluation, laboratory tests, morphological imaging and tumor markers. In most cases, cancer relapse is suggested by an increase in the serum tumor marker, while morphological imaging modalities may remain negative for a long time. In the presence of increased marker and negative or inconclusive conventional imaging, FDG PET study is frequently able to find areas of locoregional relapse or distant metastasis, thus changing the clinical management in a large number of patients. The usefulness of FDG PET has been reported for a number of tumors, including breast, ovarian, testicle, non small cell lung cancer, melanoma, head and neck, pancreas, esophagus, stomach, colo-rectal and others. Therefore, in all these tumors the follow up approach frequently includes clinical and conventional radiological procedures, as well as laboratory data. In cases of discordance or inconclusive findings, FDG PET has to be proposed for identifying early recurrent cancer.

Only recently and for few malignancies (lymphoma, colo-rectal) FDG PET has been suggested as a systematic tool in follow-up.

Treatment Planning

As with other imaging procedures, PET influences further decisions in patient management, i.e. by proper staging and relapse identification. However there are therapies that exploit PET to improve the results, such as intensity-modulated radiotherapy (IMRT). This method carries the potential benefit of increasing the therapeutic ratio by minimizing the dose delivered to nontarget tissue, with the potential of dose escalation to cancer tissue. Although computed tomography remains the gold standard of anatomic image acquisition for the purpose of target volume definition and dose calculation in radiotherapy treatment planning, FDG-PET can be usefully applied for volume definition.

Bone

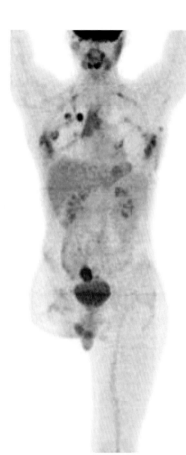

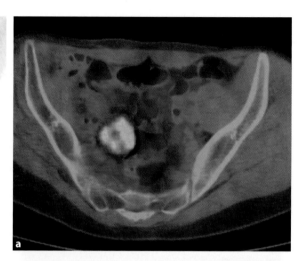

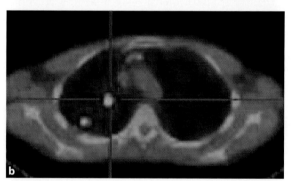

◘ PET findings

hypermetabolic pelvic mass (a) attributable to large adenopathy and two right lung nodules (b); other sites of increased uptake are evident (thymus, bilateral ribs) not related to cancer

Teaching point

PET is superior to CI concerning the correct detection of lymph node involvement and bone metastasis, whereas CT is more reliable than FDG-PET in depicting lung metastases.

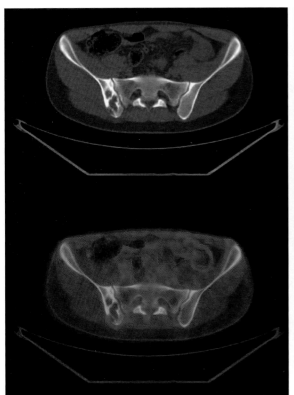 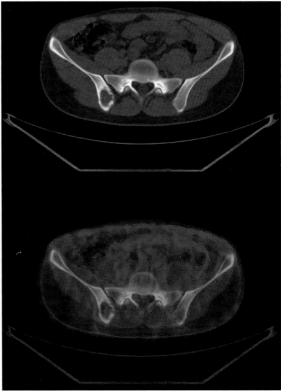

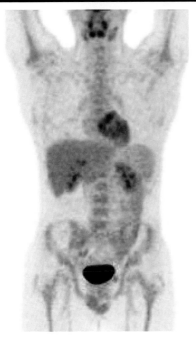

◙ PET findings

no area of increased uptake

Teaching point

PET is superior to CI concerning the evaluation of residual active disease; in any case a strict follow-up is mandatory.

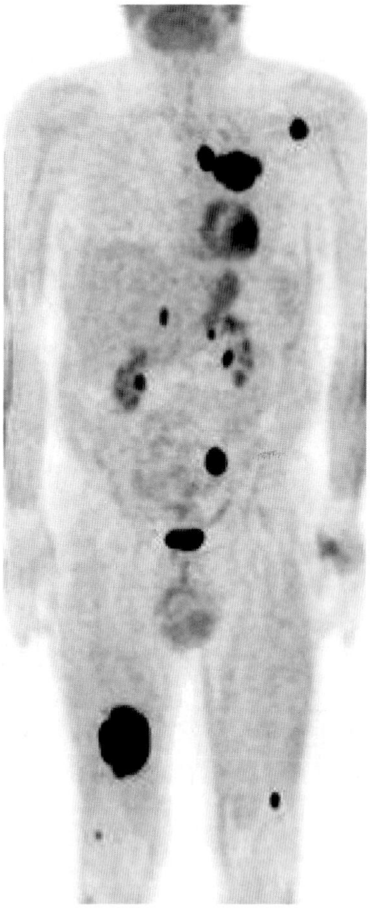

PET scan

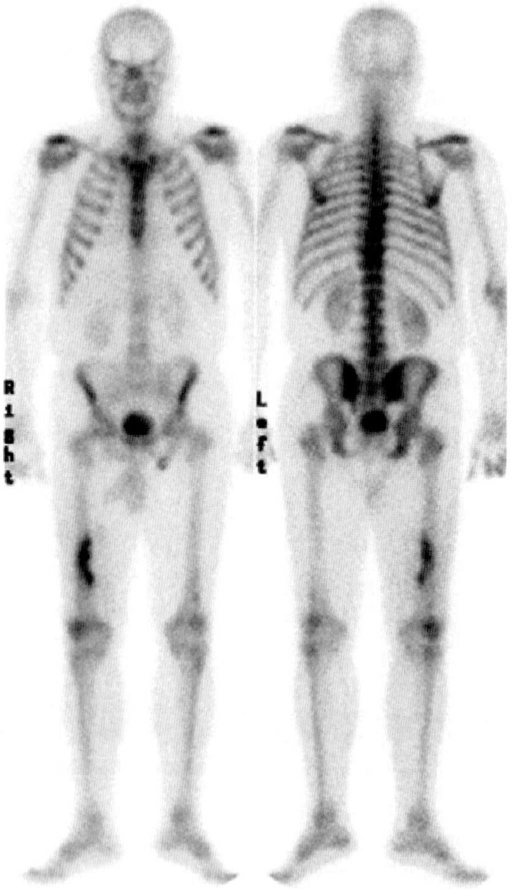

Bone scan

PET findings

several areas of increased uptake at primary lesion, lymph nodes, bilateral adrenal glands and at bone level (secondary lesions). Bone scintigraphy revealed only one lesion

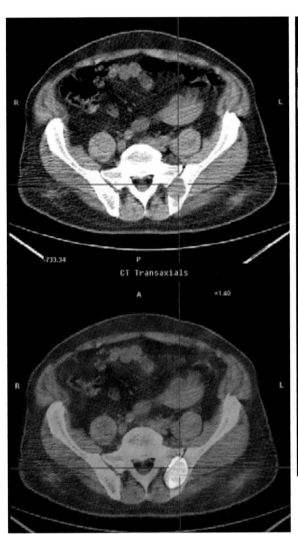

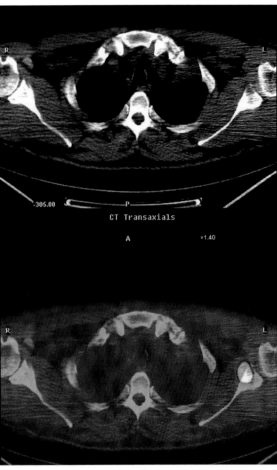

Teaching point

PET is frequently superior to conventional imaging for the identification of bone lesions.

Brain

▣ FDG PET findings

increased uptake area at right frontal lobe, suggestive of high grade malignant lesion

Teaching point

The use of FDG PET scan for grading CNS lesions is becoming less frequent; nonetheless, the degree of uptake of FDG remains predictive of tumor grade.

¹¹C-METH

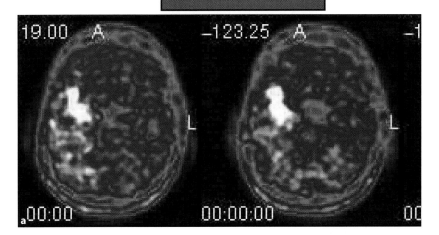

◘ **11C methionine PET findings (a)**

increased uptake area at right temporal lobe, attributable to recurrence, then confirmed at follow-up

¹⁸F-FDG

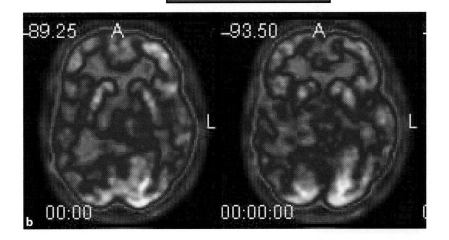

◘ **FDG PET findings (b)**

area of decreased uptake, no sign of relapse

Teaching point

FDG PET can frequently fail to early detect the presence of CNS tumor relapse, especially in low-grade tumors. 11C-methionine PET is more accurate.

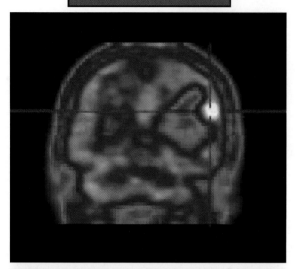

11C-METH

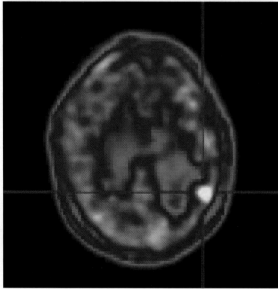

◼ **11C methionine PET findings**

increased uptake area at left temporal lobe, attributable to local recurrence

Teaching point

11C-methionine PET is useful in the differentiation of local tumor recurrence from radiation injury (scar).

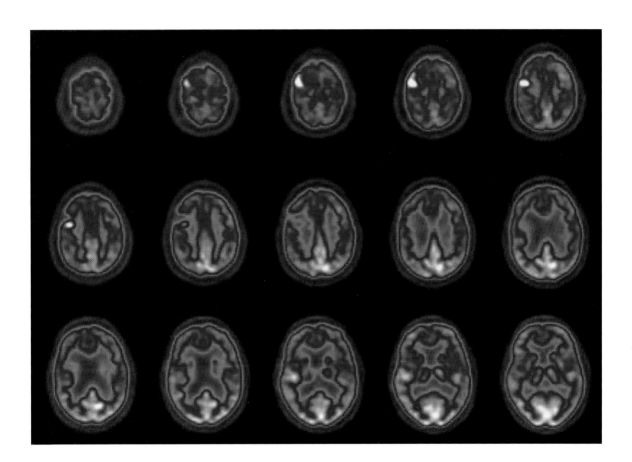

◘ FDG PET findings

increased uptake area at right frontal lobe, next to operated area, attributable to local recurrence

Teaching point

Even if FDG may be inferior to other PET tracers to demonstrate relapse of CNS tumors, a positive FDG scan in high grade cancer is highly sensitive to diagnose recurrence.

Breast

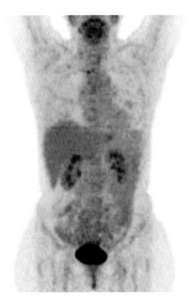

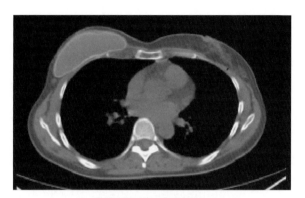

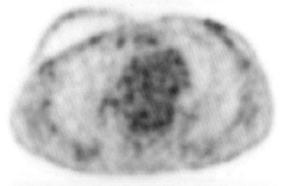

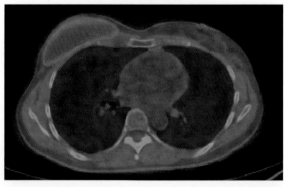

◨ PET findings

absence of uptake at the axillary lymph node

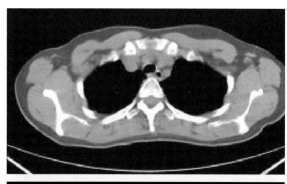

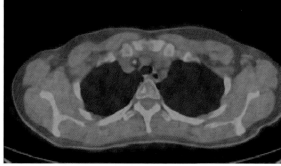

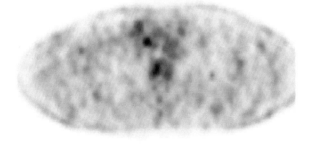

◻ PET findings

small hypermetabolic internal mammary lymph node

Teaching point

Metabolic imaging provided by FDG PET can detect tissue behavior determining potential relapse without volume alterations.

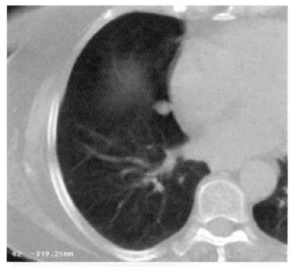 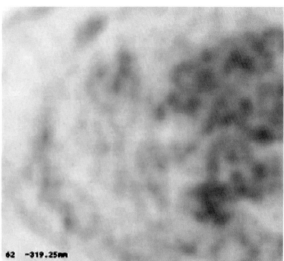

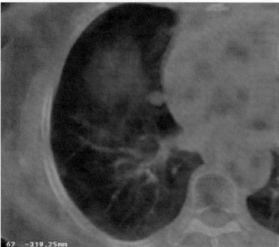

🔹 Left mastectomy for breast cancer. Post-operative CT shows a suspected secondarism at the medium lobe of right lung.

🔹 **PET findings**

no pathologic uptake corresponding to the lung lesion. Nevertheless FDG PET-CT shows one hypermetabolic left parasternal lymph node attributable to a metastasis

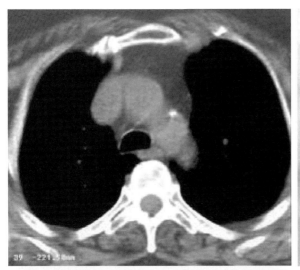
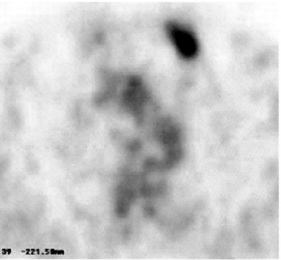
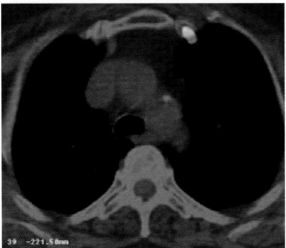

Teaching point

Early diagnosis of recurrent breast cancer is crucial to selection of the most appropriate therapy. PET/CT compared with CT has been reported to have a higher sensitivity and specificity.

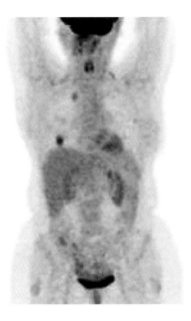

◘ PET findings

hypermetabolism of the known lung lesions. The degree of uptake is more intense at suspect lesion (SUV = 6.3) and consistent with secondary nodule. At CT follow-up only this lesion was confirmed to be neoplastic

Teaching point

Despite the good accuracy, PET does not allow for a final diagnosis. In challenging cases with several lesions of possibly different natures, PET can be helpful to make a diagnosis and even to decide therapy. However, in cases of necessary pathologic diagnosis a biopsy may be required.

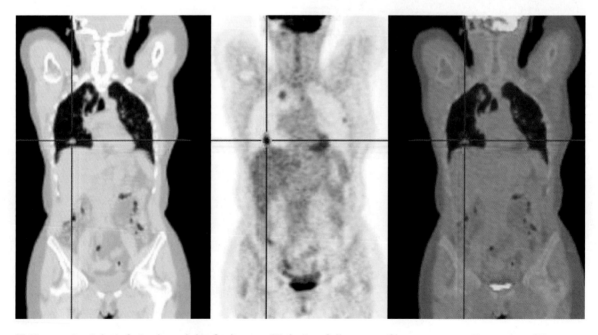

◘ Uncertain right inferior lung lobe finding at CT during follow-up of breast cancer. Two other CT findings at superior right lobe and left lobe, likely inflammatory

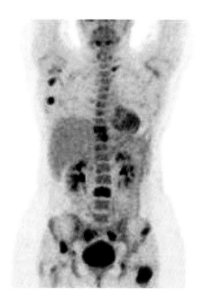

Teaching point

In breast cancer staging, PET is inferior to conventional imaging for T staging, and to sentinel node scintigraphy for N staging. However, PET can be useful in selected cases for M, enabling one to detect distant metastatic lesions.

◘ PET findings

hypermetabolic right breast lesion, ipsilateral axillary lymph nodes and several bone lesions

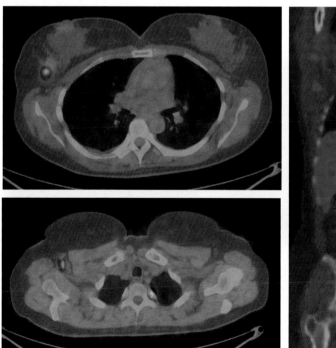

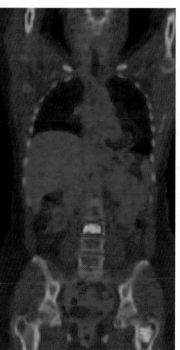

129

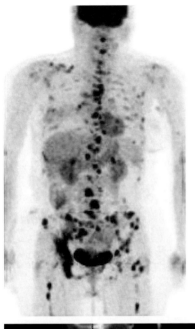

Teaching point

Despite the impressive PET finding, CT was almost negative.

■ PET findings

a number of lesions, mainly located at bone level

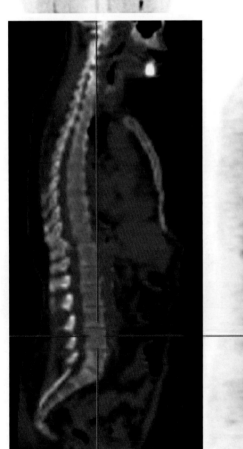

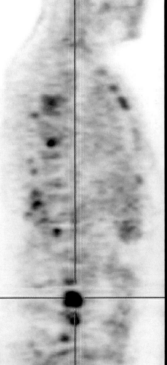

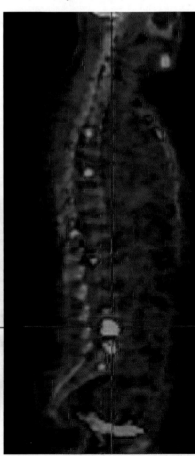

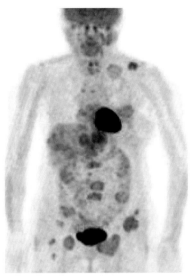

◘ PET findings

faint increased glucose activity at bone (a), liver (b) and paratracheal level, consistent with metastasis

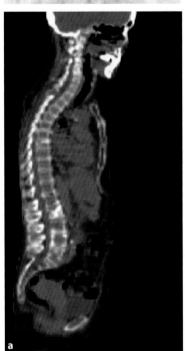

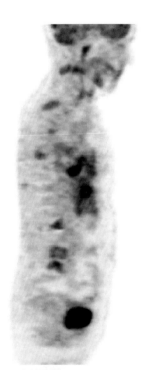

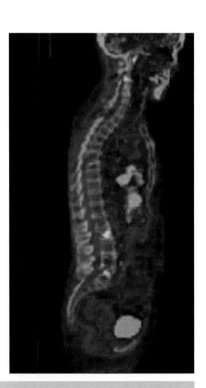

Teaching point

In old cachectic patients metastatic lesions could have a relatively low degree of FDG uptake.

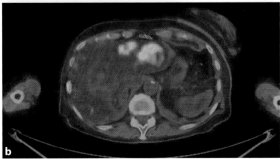

4

Case 7   **Breast Cancer. Staging (a) and Post-therapy PET (b)**

Female 35 yo

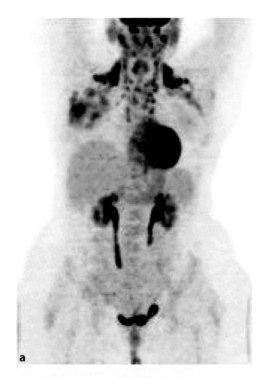 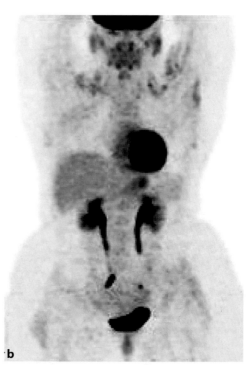

◼ Staging (a) and post-therapy PET (b)

◼ **FDG findings**

Staging PET shows the right breast lesion and hypermetabolic ipsilateral axillary lymph nodes (a,c). Complete response after surgery and chemotherapy (b,d). Brown fat is visible in both scans, more evident at presentation

Case 7   Breast Cancer. Staging (a) and Post-therapy PET (b)

4

Female 35 yo

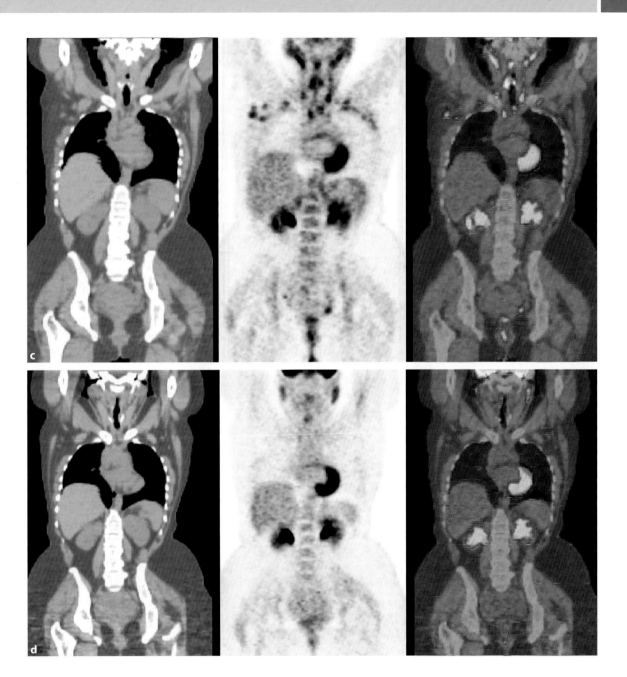

Teaching point

The presence of brown fat could hide pathologic lesions (false negative) or, on the contrary, not be correctly interpreted (false positive).

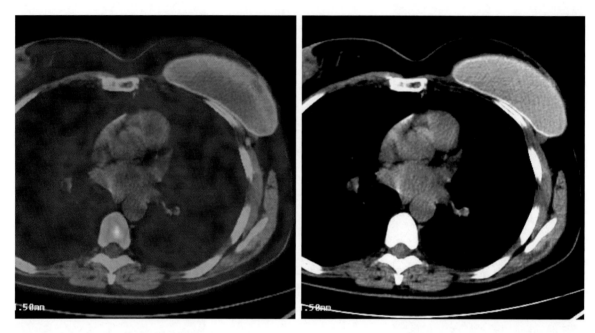

🔲 Left mastectomy for breast cancer. Follow-up CT shows a small nodule just below the prosthesis

🔲 **PET findings**

increased uptake corresponding to the lesion

Teaching point

In presence of indeterminate CT finding PET is extremely useful to confirm the suspicion of recurrence.

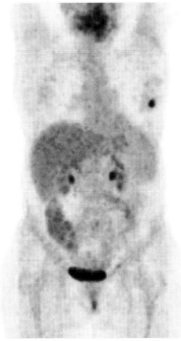

◘ PET findings

increased uptake at lesion, no other sites of hypermetabolism

Teaching point

PET is usually not used for characterizing breast lesion: however in selected cases it can provide useful information.

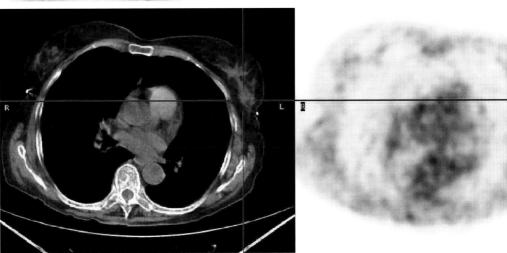

◘ Indeterminate breast lesion at mammography; inconclusive US and MR

Colo-Rectal

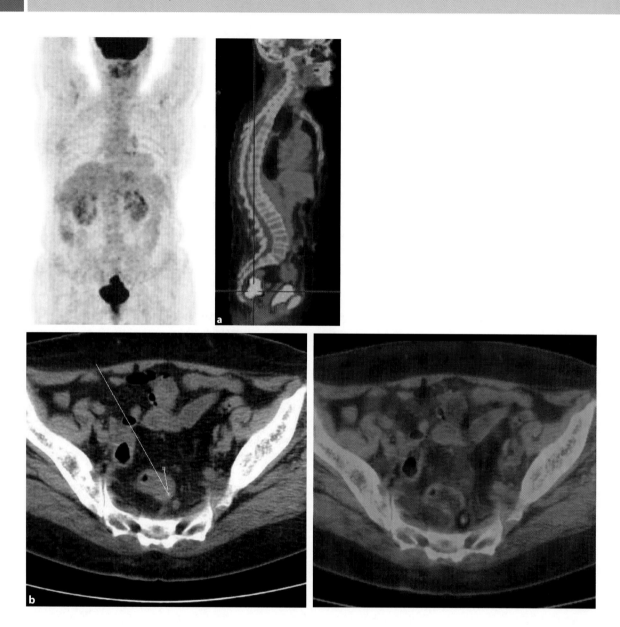

◘ PET findings

area of increased uptake at the primary lesion (a)
and small lymph node (b)

Teaching point

In patients with colorectal cancer PET can be
used to stage the disease, even if it cannot be
considered mandatory. In most cases SUV at
presentation is quite high.

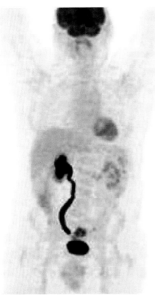

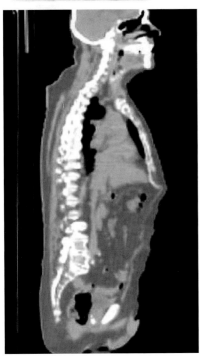

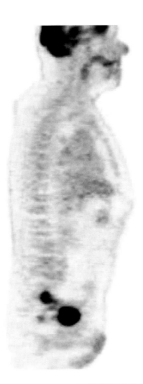

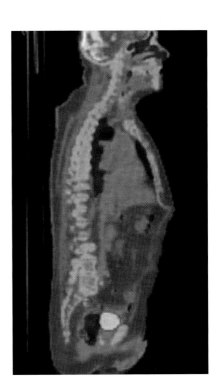

⬛ PET findings

area of increased uptake in the presacral area,
consistent with local relapse

Teaching point

In patients already operated on for colorectal
cancer PET can be helpful to discern post-
surgical scar from local relapse.

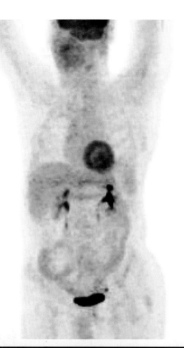
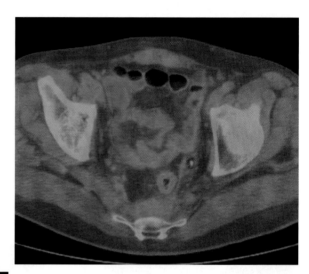
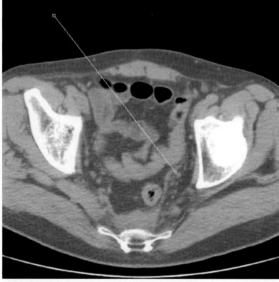
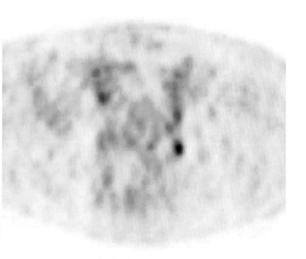

🔲 Already treated by surgery for colorectal adenocarcinoma; during follow-up increase of CEA

🔲 PET findings

small area of increased uptake in the presacral area, consistent with nodal disease

Teaching point

In patients already operated for colorectal cancer PET is particularly helpful when a relapse is suspected and other imaging methods are negative or inconclusive.

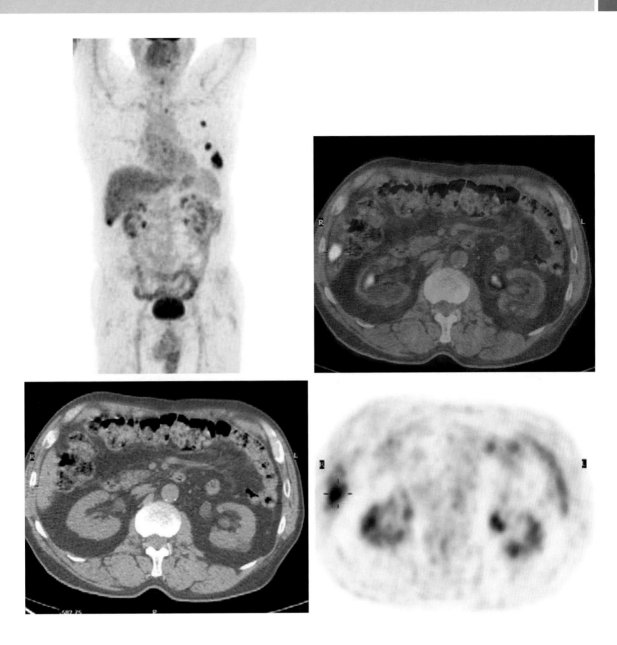

◘ PET findings

several lesions at the left lung, small lesion at liver

Teaching point

In patients already operated on for colorectal cancer PET is extremely useful in cases of suspected relapse.

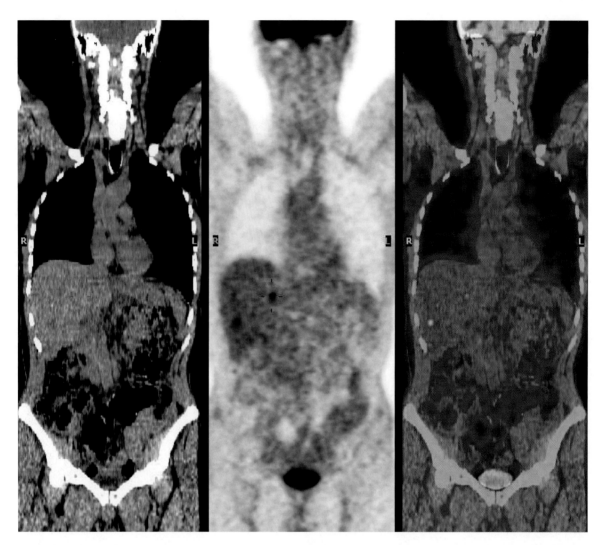

🔲 Rectal adenocarcinoma resected by surgery. Post-operative increasing of CA 19-9. Conventional imaging (US, CT, MRI) was negative

🔲 PET findings

small hepatic metastases

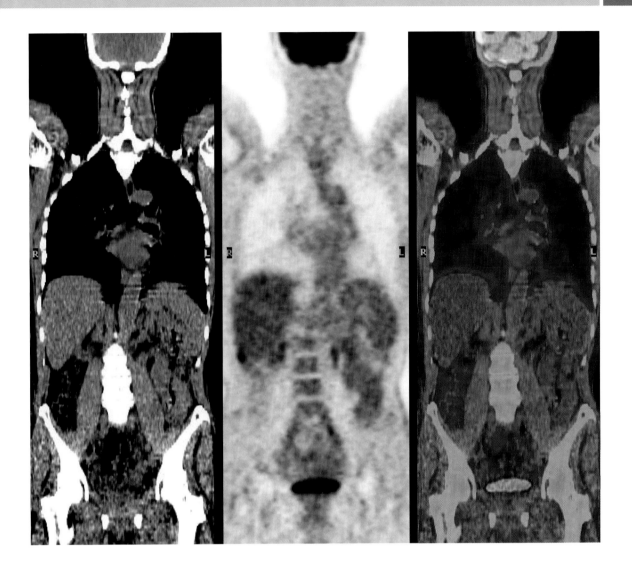

Teaching point

PET/CT has been reported to be more accurate in the detection of liver metastasis compared with CT alone; the cost and availability of the two methods have to be taken into account for clinical flow charts. Data regarding ultrasonography and SPIO-enhanced MR are less conclusive; nonetheless, it can be stated that FDG PET can have a relevant role in the evaluation of doubtful liver findings.

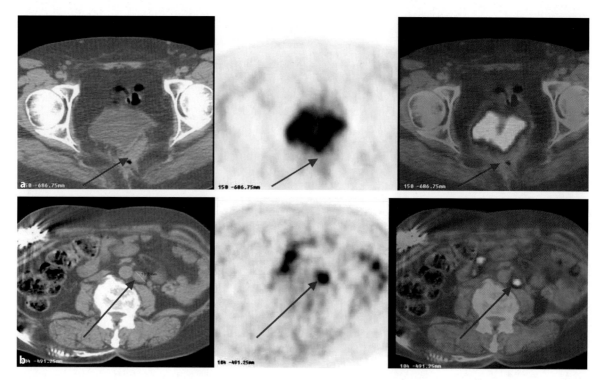

■ Previous sigmoidectomy for adenocarcinoma; recent CEA increase (80.0 ng/ml) CT: mass behind the urinary bladder suspected for relapse.

■ **PET findings**

no evidence of pathologic uptake behind the bladder (a). Presence of a hypermetabolic para-aortic lymph adenopathy (b)

Teaching point

PET/CT sensitivity for the assessment of distant metastasis of colorectal cancer is very high (> 90%) and probably better than MR and CT.

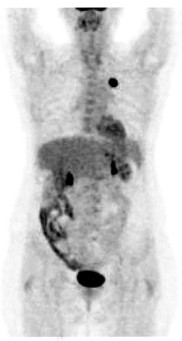

◘ PET findings

single lesion at the left lung, no evidence of other pathologic areas

Teaching point

After demonstration of a relapse, PET is accurate for restaging the patient. The exclusion of other metastasis enables surgical or radiotherapy approach to the lung lesions.

145

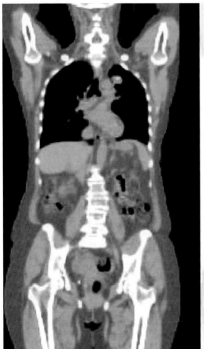
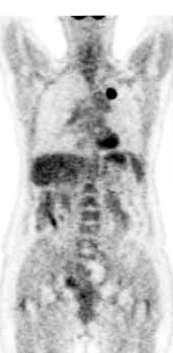
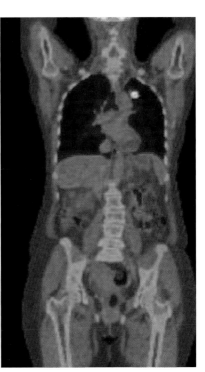

◘ Hemicolectomy for adenocarcinoma. Follow-up CT shows left lung nodule suspect for metastasis.

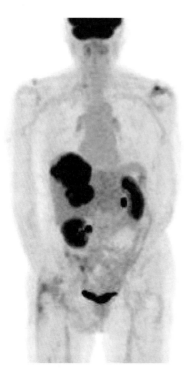

◙ Hemicolectomy for adenocarcinoma. Follow-up
CT shows right liver lobe metastasis.

◙ **PET findings**

huge hypermetabolic lesion at the right lobe. No
evidence of other pathologic areas

Teaching point

The exclusion of distant metastasis
localization enables a surgical approach
to the right liver lobe. This capacity is due
to the whole body field of view and to the
high accuracy of FDG PET. Other findings
evident in the scan are dislocation of right
kidney, arthrosis (especially at left shoulder,
for the pain patient cannot be scanned arms
up), faint uptake at both lung hilar regions:
of course, none of these findings has any
oncological relevance.

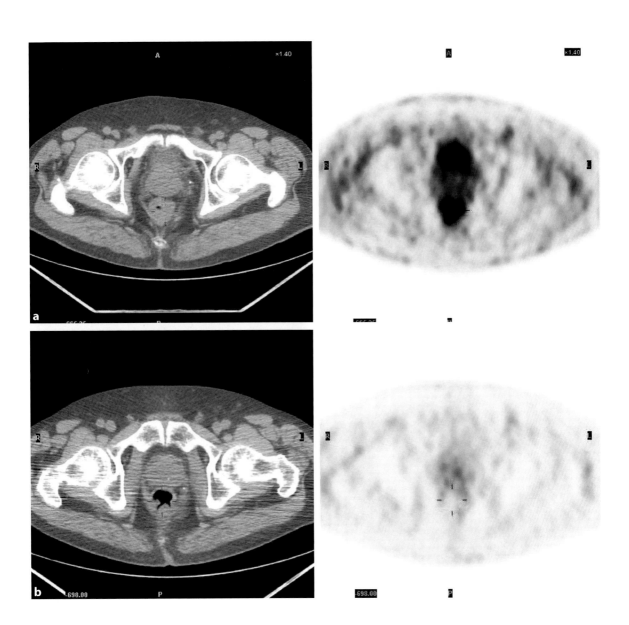

▣ PET findings

increased uptake at the known primary lesions before therapy (a), after treatment (b) complete metabolic response (SUV max from 10 to 2)

Teaching point

PET is the most accurate method to evaluate response to neoadjuvant chemotherapy + radiotherapy.

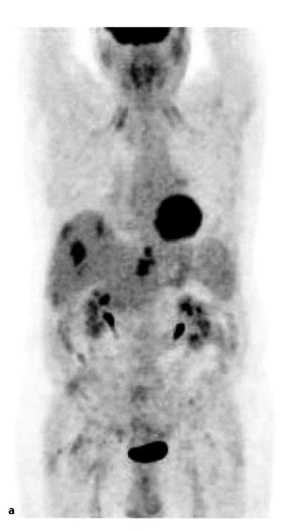

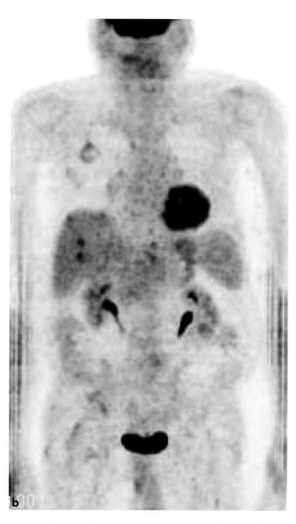

◘ PET findings

increased uptake at liver lesions and lymph nodes before therapy (a), after treatment (b) partial metabolic response of liver and nodal lesions, with appearance of a new secondary localization at right lung

Teaching point

PET can demonstrate the response to therapy, even in cases of discordant results (regression at some sites with progression in others).

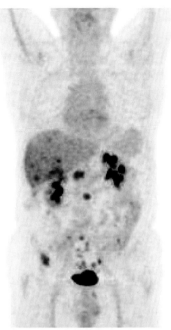

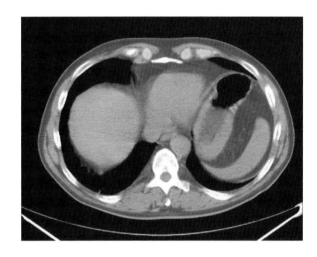

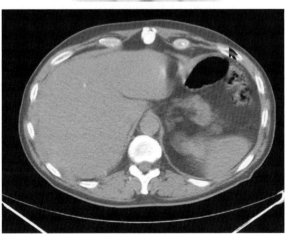

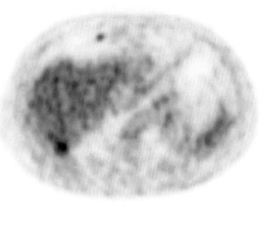

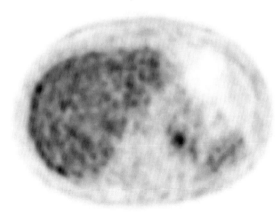

◘ PET findings

several lesions at lymph nodes and initial peritoneal carcinosis

149

Teaching point

PET may be a sensitive method to early identification of peritoneal diffusion of the disease, typically at liver capsule.

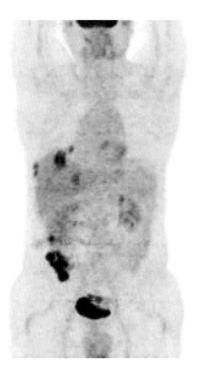

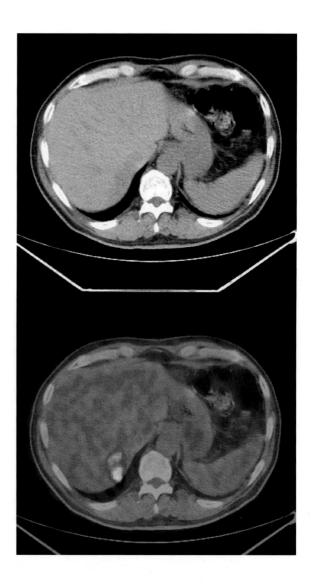

◘ PET findings

large lesion at the colon (local relapse), and
pathologic uptake at liver and lymph nodes

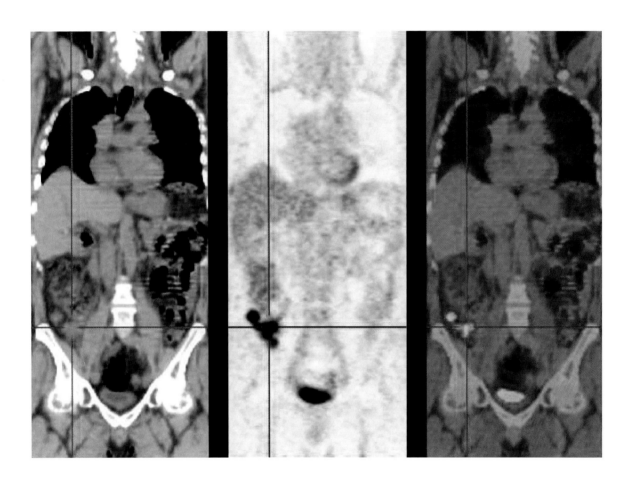

Teaching point

After demonstration of a relapse, PET is accurate for restaging the patient. PET-CT can localize local recurrence, as well as nodal and parenchymal lesions.

CUP

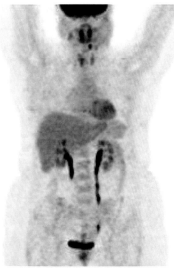

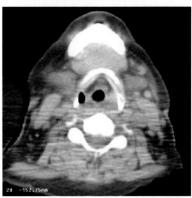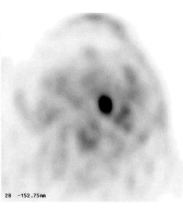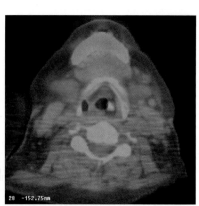

◘ The patient had a secondary lesion in one laterocervical lymph node (squamocellular carcinoma), with no detectable primary tumor after physical examination and conventional imaging tests (X-Rays, CT and US)

◘ PET findings

hypermetabolic area at left laryngeal wall. Furthermore, PET scan shows increased and diffuse FDG uptake in the thyroid parenchyma

Teaching point

PET and PET/CT can help localize the primary in CUP in a range of 20–50% of cases. Also, PET can be useful for detecting unsuspected distant disease, especially in patients with undifferentiated nodal histological findings.

Case 2   Familiar with Colorectal Cancer. Negative Colonoscopy but Increased CEA

4

Male 72 yo

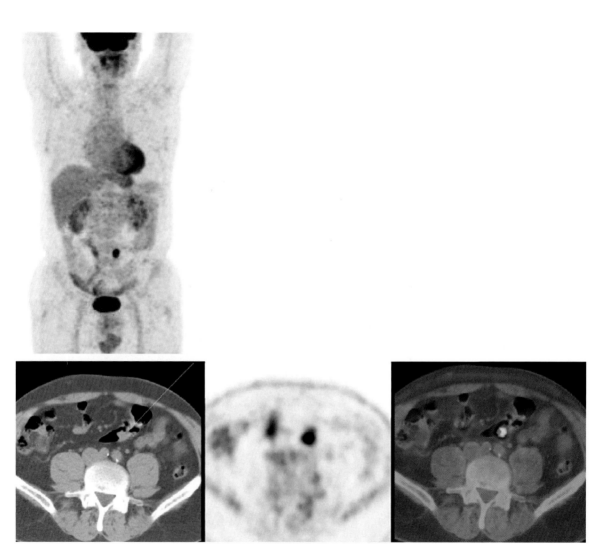

◘ Familiar with colorectal cancer. Negative colonoscopy but increased CEA. PET is performed to search an hypothetic lesion.

4

Case 2   Familiar with Colorectal Cancer. Negative Colonoscopy but Increased CEA

Male 72 yo

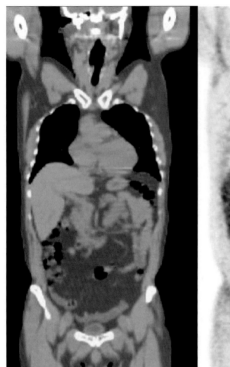 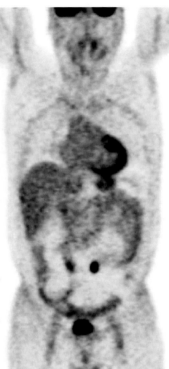 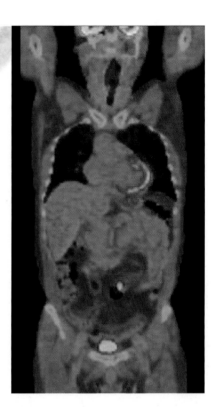

🔲 PET findings

one hypermetabolic endoluminal intestinal lesion at the mesogaster. Following histopathology confirm malignity of small bowel lesion.

Teaching point

Endoscopy methods are not able to explore for its larger part the small bowel. PET could find and set the potential malignancy of an intestinal lesion.

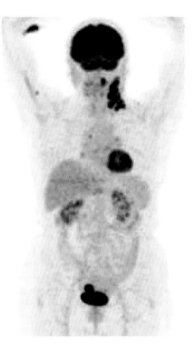 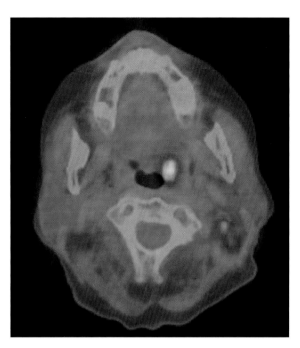

◘ Patient presented with swollen left laterocervical lymph nodes

◘ **PET findings**

hypermetabolic area at left oropharingeal wall (primary tumor), and at many lymph nodes

Teaching point

The usefulness of PET in CUP is related to its capability in identifying cancers of very different location and origin.

Esophageal

4

Case 1   **Pre-operatory Evaluation of Esophageal Cancer. CT staging: N0 M0**

Male 72 yo

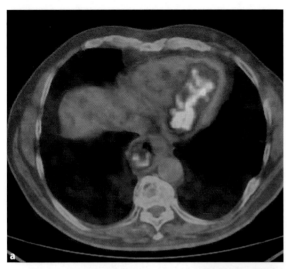

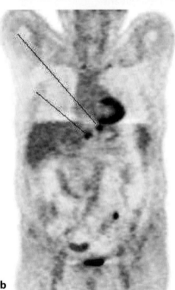
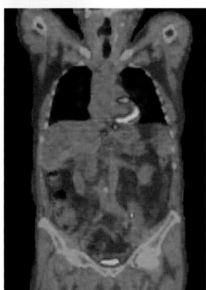

▣ PET findings

primary lesion (a) and hypermetabolic lymph nodes at paraesophageal and phrenic level (b)

Teaching point

There is no algorithm for the initial staging of esophageal cancer that could definitely be considered standard of care. The addition of FDG-PET to EUS and CT offers little information to the initial treatment stratification of patients. However, in patients with doubtful EUS, FDG-PET may have some clinical utility, especially for N and M staging.

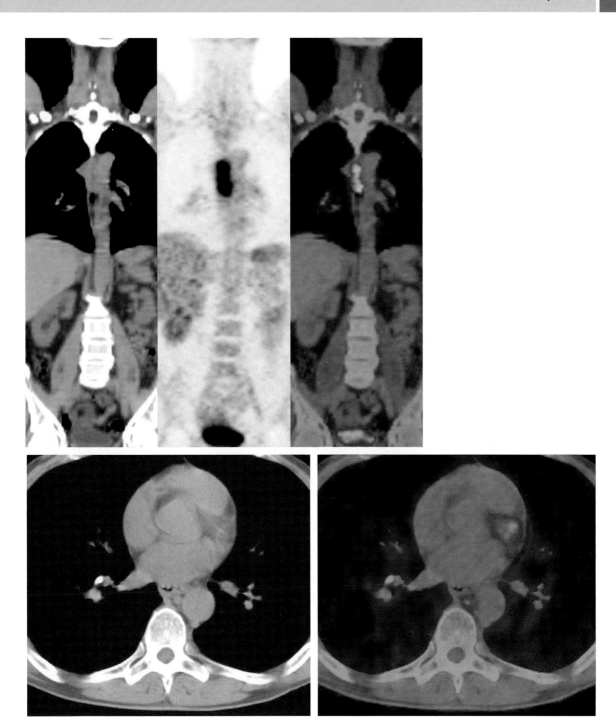

▣ PET findings

increased uptake at primary lesion and small
lymph node

Teaching point

PET can identify involved nodes (N +)
negative at CT.

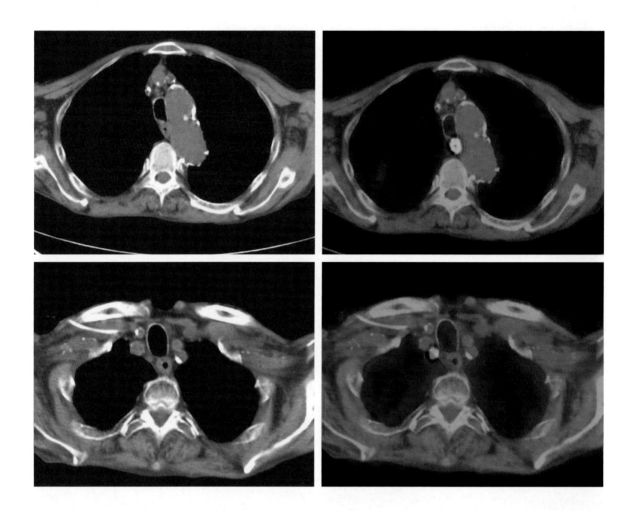

■ PET findings

increased uptake at primary lesion and small lymph node

Teaching point

PET can identify involved nodes (N +) negative at CT.

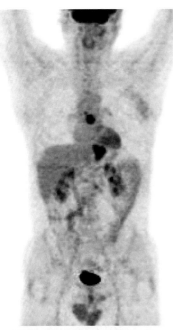

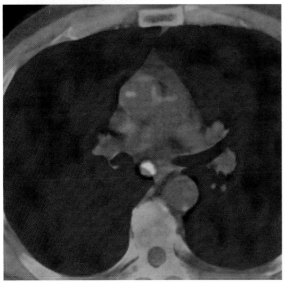

▣ PET findings

increased uptake at primary lesion and lymph nodes

Teaching point

PET can usefully be employed for N and M staging of esophageal cancer.

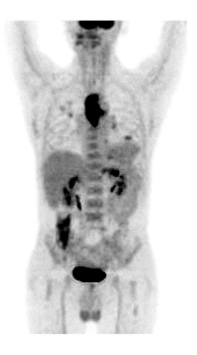

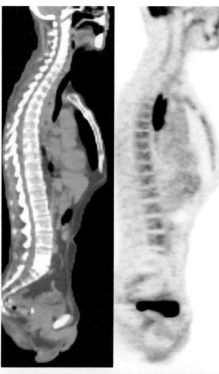

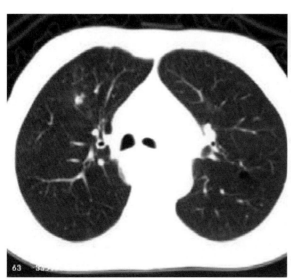

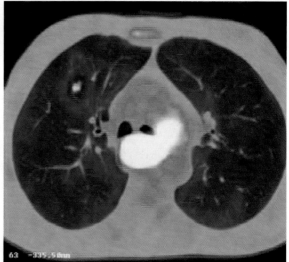

◘ PET findings

wide lesion with intense FDG uptake and lung secondary lesions

Teaching point

Distant metastases are not infrequent at presentation of esophageal cancer, and PET is helpful to show their presence.

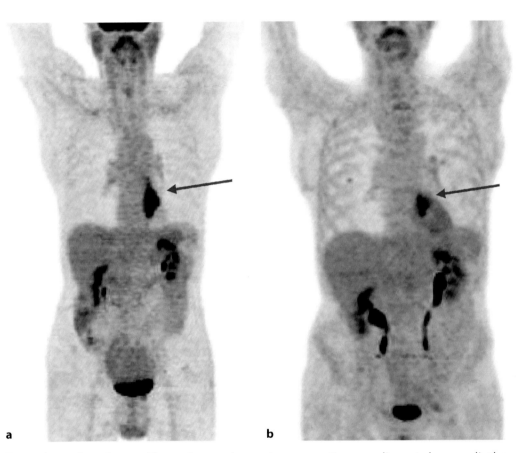

◘ Esophageal carcinoma. The patient underwent preoperative neoadjuvant chemoradiotherapy.

a   b

◘ PET findings

Staging PET (a) shows the hypermetabolic lesion (SUVmax = 11) Six months later, after 6 cycles of neoadjuvant chemoradiotherapy, PET shows a decrease of FDG uptake (SUVmax = 6)

Teaching point

FDG-PET standardized uptake value (SUV) may be predictive of the response of esophageal carcinoma patients to preoperative chemoradiotherapy Esophagectomy should still be considered even if the post-therapy FDG-PET scan is normal because microscopic residual disease cannot be ruled out.

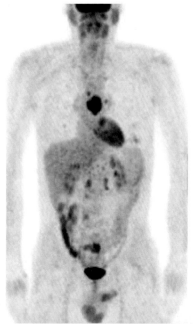

◘ PET findings

documentation of local (a) and distant (b: lymph nodes; c: lung lesion) all consistent with relapse

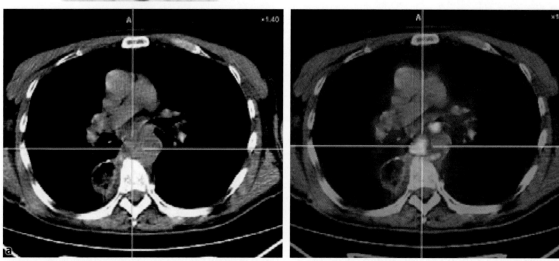

◘ Previous surgical treatment for esophageal carcinoma. During follow-up, CT scan shows a lesion suspected for local relapse.

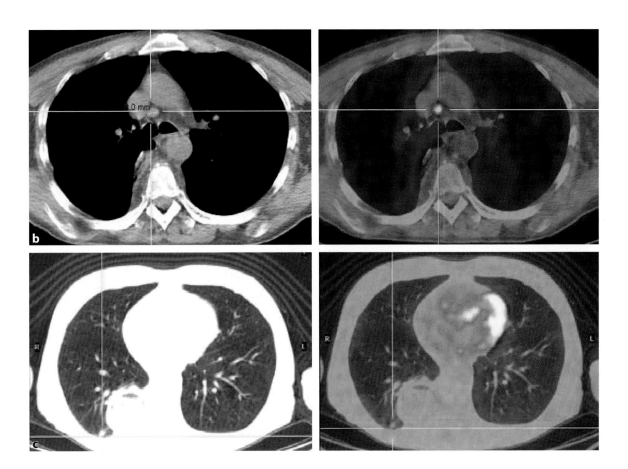

Teaching point

In the diagnosis of recurrent oesophageal carcinoma, the sensitivity of FDG-PET is higher than that of CT in detecting locoregional recurrence, but its specificity has been reported to be lower; in distant organs the sensitivity of PET in detecting metastasis is higher, apart from lung lesions.

Gastric and Small Bowel

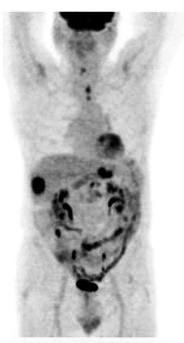

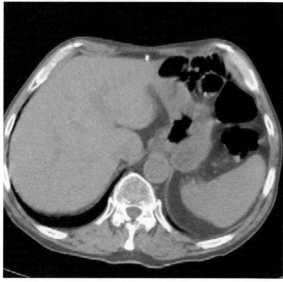

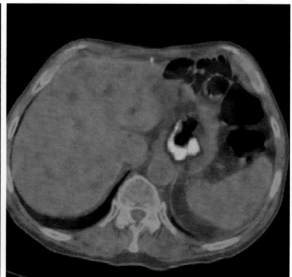

◘ PET findings

hypermetabolic areas at gastric level, local and
distant lymph nodes, and one large liver lesion

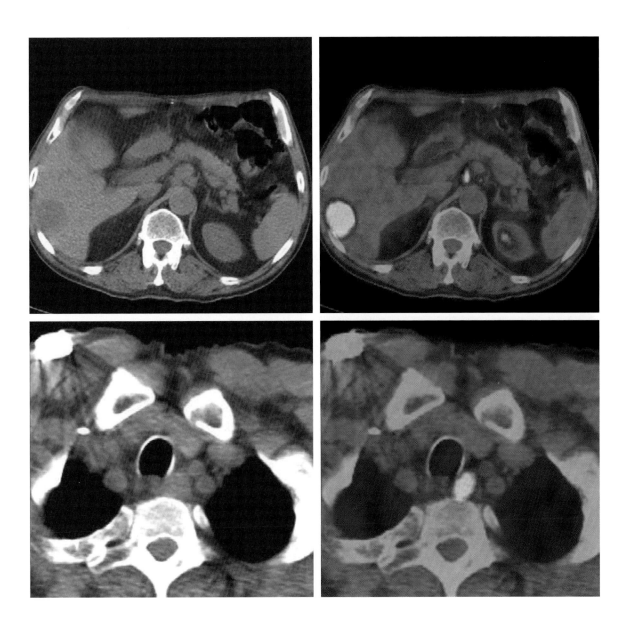

Teaching point

FDG PET is not frequently used for staging gastric cancer; in selected cases, however, can be helpful to establish the surgical approach.

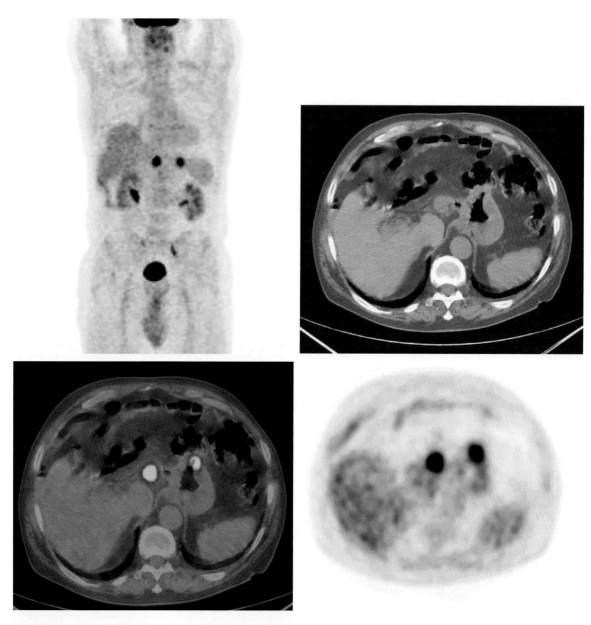

◘ Gastric cancer treated by surgery and chemotherapy. At follow-up suspect nodal relapse.

◘ PET findings

one hypermetabolic area at gastro-jejunal anastomosis and one celiac hypermetabolic adenopathy

Teaching point

Surgical scar could sometimes hide an area of local recurrence of disease because of anatomic distortion.

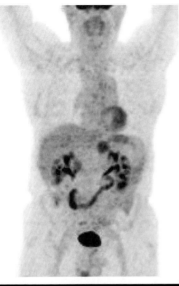

⬛ Previous radical gastrectomy for a gastric cancer. Two years later weight loss with negative ecotomography and endoscopy.

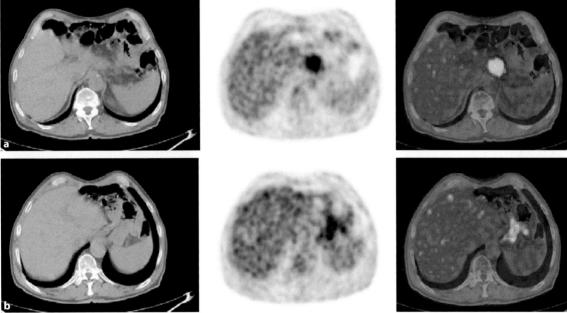

173

⬛ **PET findings**

relapse at one peripancreatic lymph node (a) and at the gastric stump (b)

Teaching point

Although tumor recurrence has a poor prognosis, early identification is helpful because it may allow patients with minimal adenopathy or small recurrent masses to respond better to chemotherapy or radiation therapy.

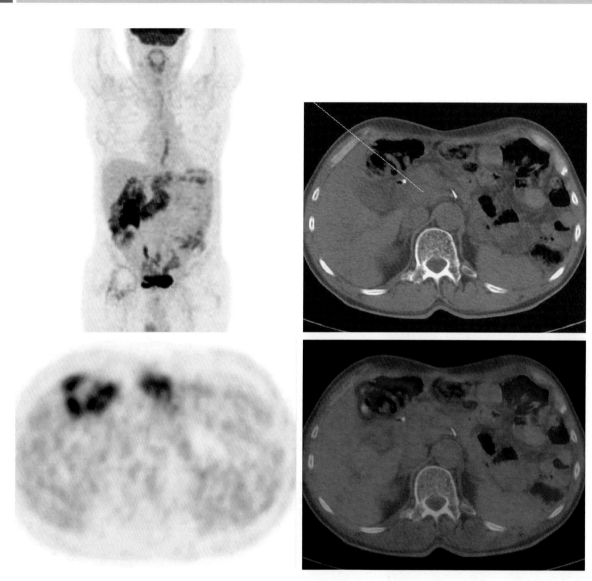

■ Gastric carcinoma operated on and subsequently treated with chemotherapy. CT revealed an expansive mass at the liver hilum.

■ **PET findings**

lack of uptake at the abdominal mass. Urinary stasis at the right kidney. Follow-up proves the mass was a post-surgical fibrotic tissue

Teaching point

CT is the primary tool for the investigation of suspected recurrence due to its widespread availability and relatively low cost, but often cannot help in discerning treatment-induced morphologic changes from tumor recurrence.

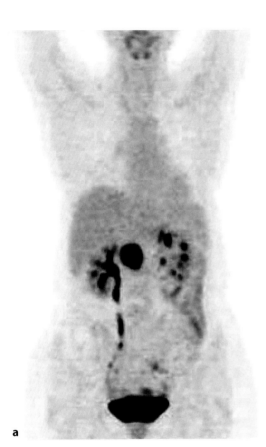
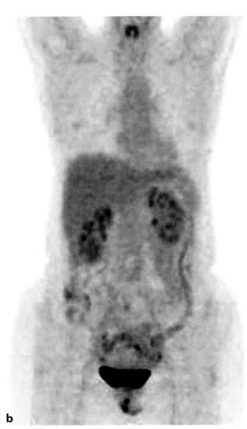

a

b

◘ PET findings

increased FDG uptake of gastric tumor before therapy (a). After 40 days, PET images show a complete response (b)

Teaching point

Molecular imaging is considered at present to be the most useful tool for early evaluation of response to therapy because it provides information on tumor viability. This approach can be applied to most solid cancers.

Female 67 yo

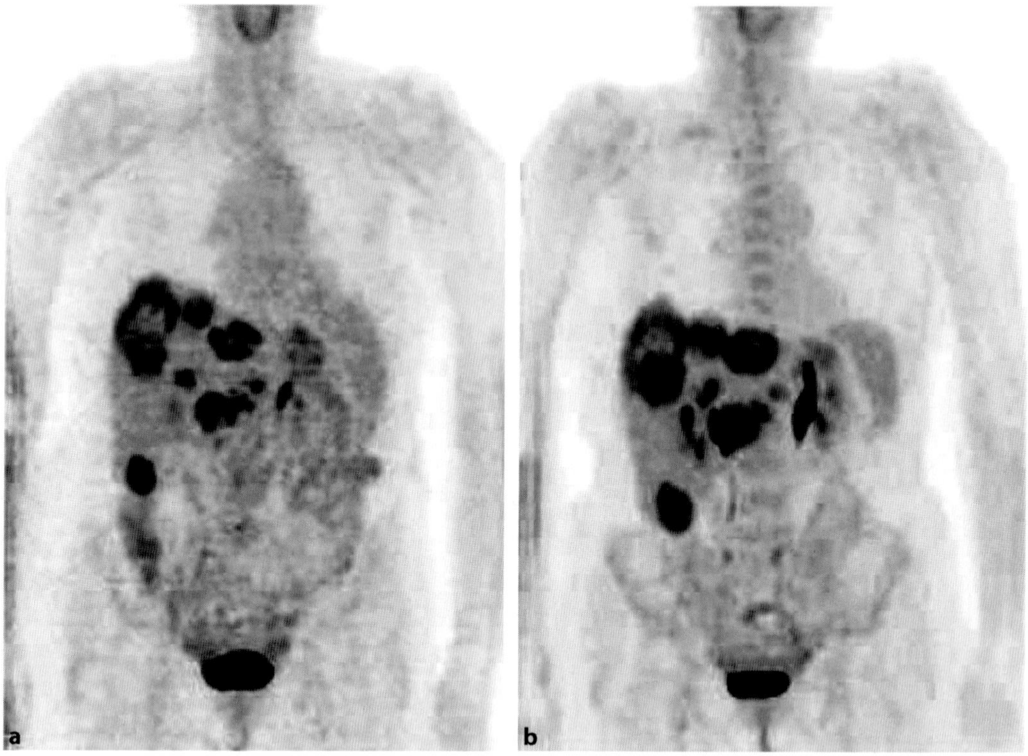

PET findings

multiple hypermetabolic hepatic lesions and inter-aorto-caval adenopathy (a). After 43 days, post-therapy scan shows a very faint decrease of FDG uptake, but size enlargement of some lesions (b). Stable/progressive disease

Teaching point

For early evaluation of response to therapy, EORTC criteria are employed, allowing one to categorize patients as complete responders, partial responders, stable disease or progression.

Gynecology

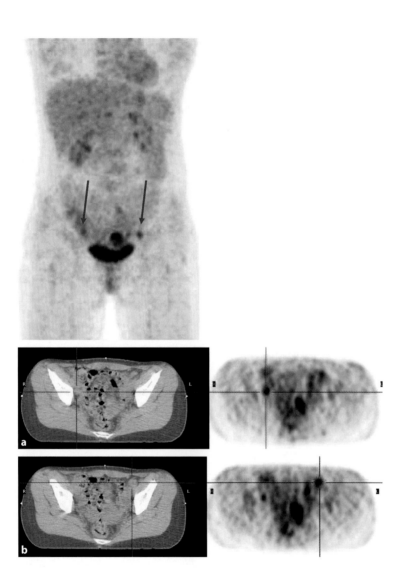

◘ PET findings

increased FDG uptake at the uterine lesion and at two bilateral iliac lymph nodes (red arrows and a,b) consistent with metastasis

Teaching point

FDG-PET can sometimes provide crucial information in the pre-treatment staging procedure in patients with uterine cancer.

Case 2   Uterine Cervical Carcinoma After Therapy. Follow-up PET

4

Female 74 yo

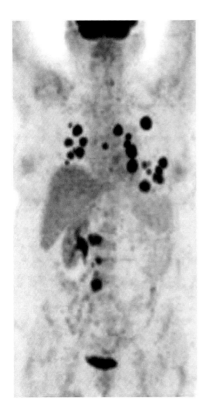

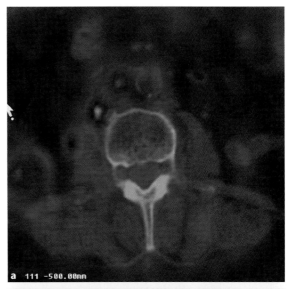

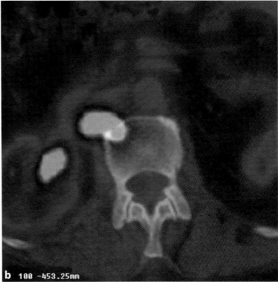

179

◘ PET findings

multiple hypermetabolic lesions at lung parenchyma, mediastinal and right iliac lymph nodes (a) with bone involvement (b). All findings are consistent with recurrent disease

Teaching point

An accurate restaging (allowed by whole body field of view) could avoid wrong treatment (such as surgical metastasectomy).

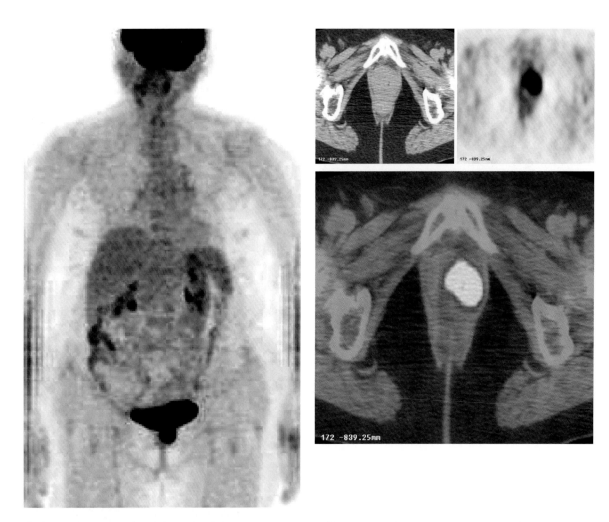

🔲 Cervical cancer after bilateral isteroannessectomy. Follow-up US shows uncertain vaginal lesion.

🔲 **PET findings**

hypermetabolism of vaginal lesion consistent with recurrent disease

Teaching point

FDG-PET scan is a sensitive post-therapy surveillance modality for detection of recurrent cervical cancer even in asymptomatic patients, and aids in deciding treatment plans and, eventually, may have favorable impact on prognosis and survival.

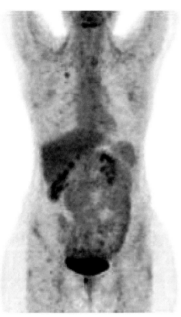

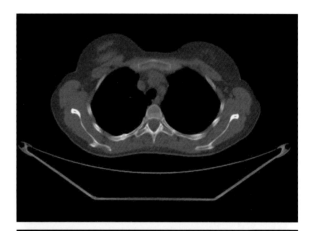

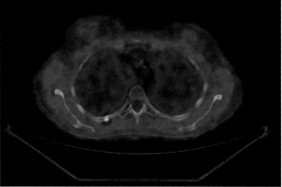

◘ Cervical cancer, at follow-up clinical identification of vaginal lesion.

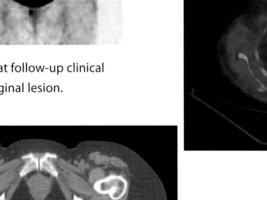

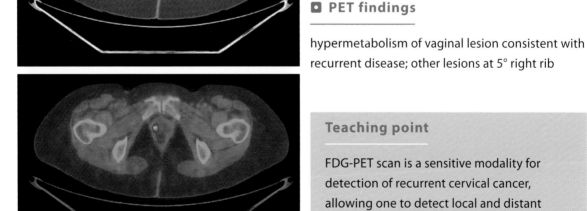

◘ **PET findings**

hypermetabolism of vaginal lesion consistent with recurrent disease; other lesions at 5° right rib

Teaching point

FDG-PET scan is a sensitive modality for detection of recurrent cervical cancer, allowing one to detect local and distant lesions.

Head and Neck

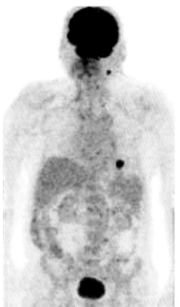

◘ PET findings

increased uptake at the rhinopharynx, one left laterocervical lymph node and one hypermetabolic left lung nodule (secondarism)

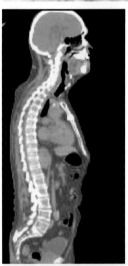
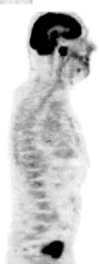
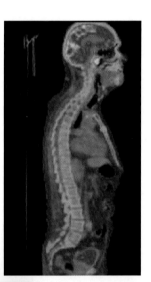

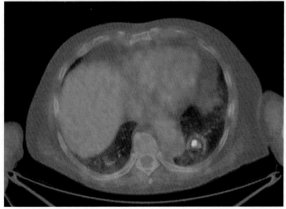

Teaching point

Detection of metastatic disease in head and neck cancer patients is crucial because patients with distant metastasis will not benefit from surgical therapy. PET imaging has been suggested to have significant potential in the detection of occult distant metastatic disease.

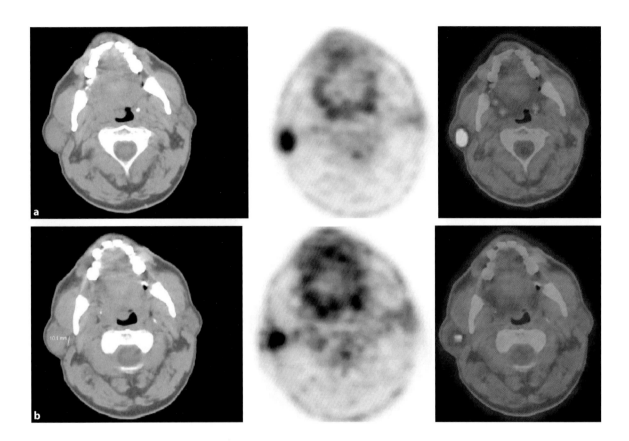

◘ PET findings

large hypermetabolic lesion in the right parotid gland (a) with lymph node at the medial side of the gland (b)

Teaching point

Head and neck carcinoma staging is very complex. This is confirmed by the significant discordance in the published literature. Clinical N0 is the most critical situation: CT, PET-CT, US, and SNB shows various accuracy values in published studies.

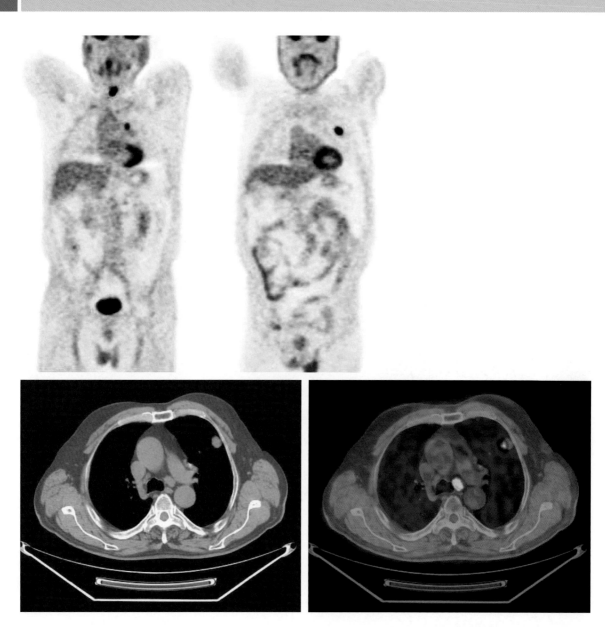

◘ PET findings

increased FDG activity of the known laryngeal lesion, at lymph nodes and at lung (N + M +), already demonstrated at CT scan

Teaching point

PET can correctly identify the primary tumor as well as nodal involvement and metastases; however in most cases CT can provide similar information at lower cost.

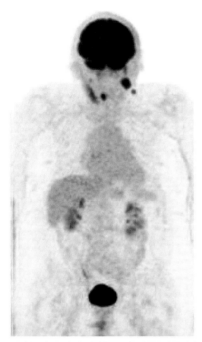

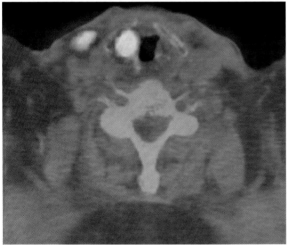

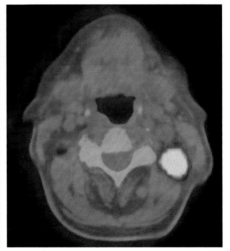

187

◘ PET findings

increased uptake at the larynx, and two left laterocervical lymph node

Teaching point

In cases of restaging, PET is also useful in detecting local and distant extension of the disease. Care has to be paid in the presence of post-surgical scars, and for the common presence of muscle contraction (as in this case). Scans have to be performed arms down.

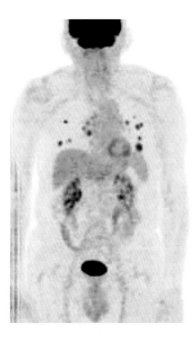

◘ Previous surgical resection of a parotid gland adenoidocystic carcinoma. During follow-up, uncertain CT findings for metastatic lung lesions.

◘ **PET findings**

several bilateral areas of increased FDG uptake consistent with secondary lung lesions

Teaching point

Some rare forms of cancer may be difficult to evaluate. PET can contribute not only to stage or document relapse, but in some cases also to clarify the nature of findings already seen by other imaging methods.

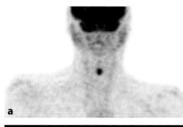

◘ Left vocal cord carcinoma. Staging (a,b) and post-neoadjuvant radiotherapy (c) PET.

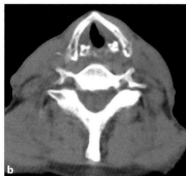
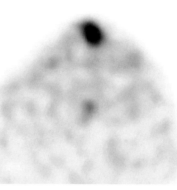
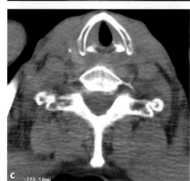
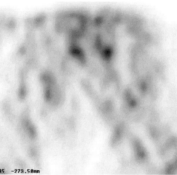

◘ PET findings

increased FDG activity of the known laryngeal lesion (a,b), after radiotherapy and before surgery treatment, PET scan is completely negative (c)

Teaching point

The development of alternative treatment regimens in clinical oncology (such as neoadjuvant therapy) has increased the need for early prediction of cancer therapy outcome, detecting patients for whom therapy will fail and avoiding significant morbidity. Data from prospective randomized studies are needed to define better the role of 18F-FDG PET in differentiating responders from nonresponders.

Lung

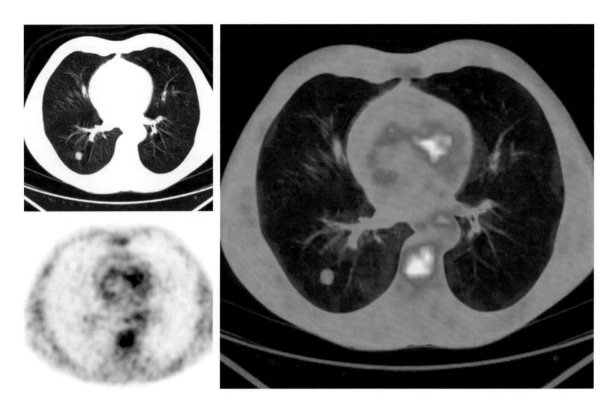

◻ No tabagism. Pre-surgical chest X-rays (for hip prosthesis) show a right solitary lung nodular opacity. CT confirmed the presence of a solitary pulmonary nodule.

◻ **PET findings**

no pathologic uptake corresponding to the lung nodule

Teaching point

Most solitary pulmonary nodules have benign causes (60–70%), especially after the introduction of multi-slice CT. PET demonstrates an excellent performance in classifying SPNs as benign or malignant, resulting in an overall significantly improved accuracy.

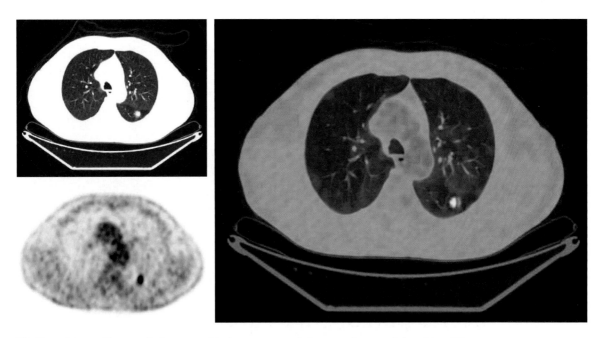

■ Chest X-rays (for persisting cough) show one nodular opacity, confirmed by CT scan.

■ **PET findings**

increased uptake at the lung nodule (SUVmax = 8)

Teaching point

Subsequent histopathology confirms the malignancy of the lesion (adenocarcinoma). In the evaluation of indeterminate pulmonary nodules, FDG PET has a very high sensitivity (> 90%) and good specificity (about 80%).

Male 77 yo

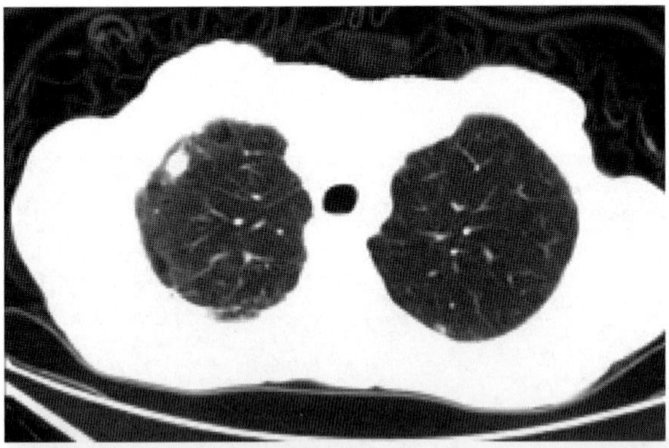

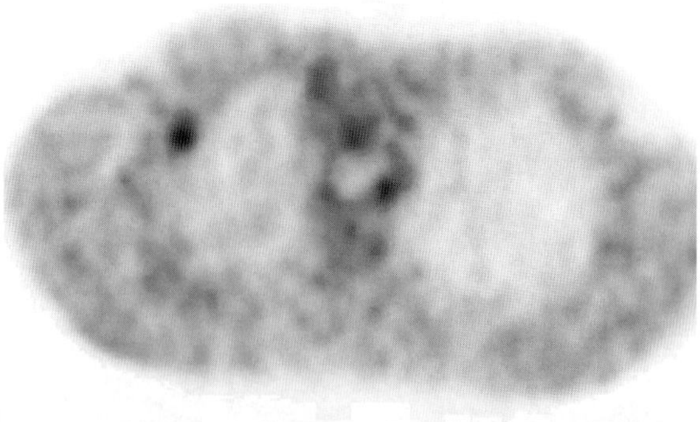

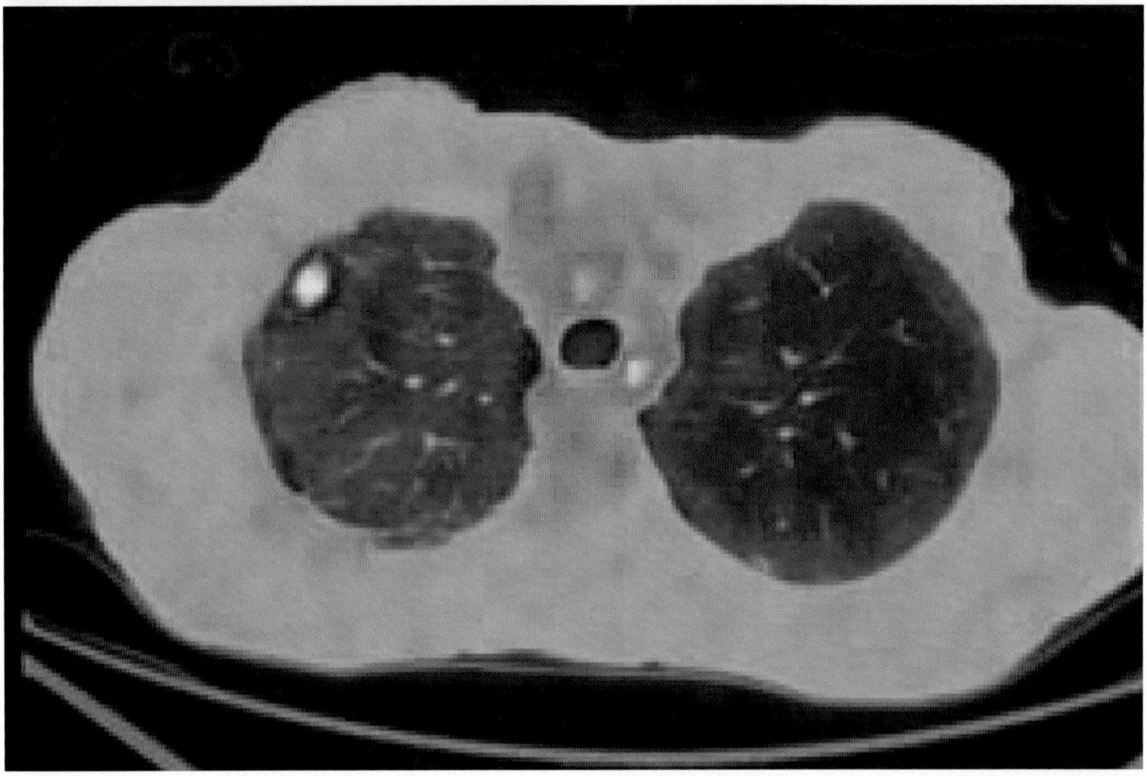

PET findings

increased uptake at the lung nodule (SUVmax = 5.4)

Teaching point

Subsequent histopathology ruled out the malignity of the lesion, revealing a sclero-calcific nodule with chronic inflammatory cells. The specificity of FDG PET is not absolute (about 80%), and false positive findings can be caused by tuberculosis, sarcoidosis and many other causes.

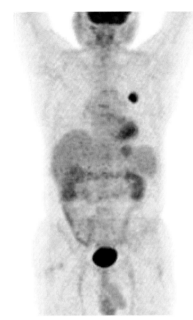

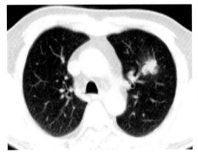 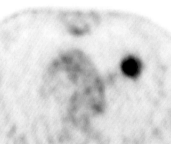 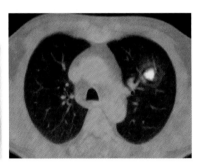

◘ PET findings

increased uptake at the known primary lesions, no other site of uptake (N0 M0). Stage confirmed at intervention

Teaching point

PET-CT is almost mandatory to properly stage a patient with non small cell lung cancer.

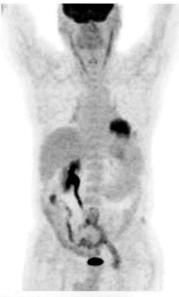

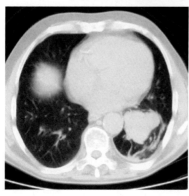 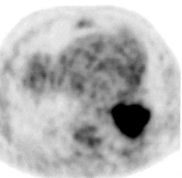 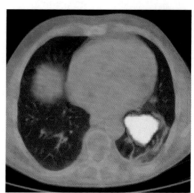

◘ PET findings

increased uptake at the known primary lesions, no other site of uptake (N0 M0)

Teaching point

Histology demonstrates an anaplastic carcinoma; despite the large dimension, stage N0 was confirmed. The faint bilateral hilar uptake was not reported and indeed has no relevance, as well as the bilateral activity in the neck, clearly attributable to muscle contraction.

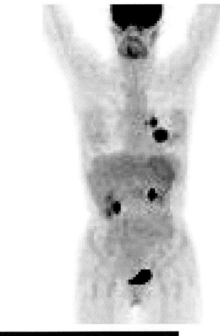

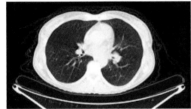 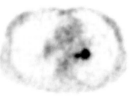 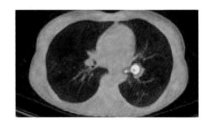

◘ PET findings

increased uptake at the known primary lesions, two other omolateral nodal sites of uptake (N1 M0)

Teaching point

Histology demonstrates an adenocarcinoma. For staging purposes it is very important to correctly identify the involved lymph nodes, and therefore the use of PET-CT is mandatory.

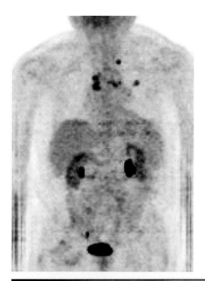

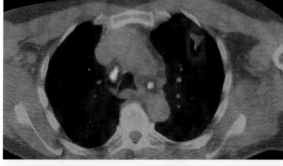

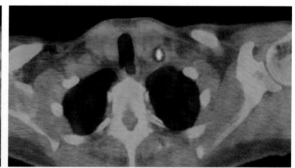

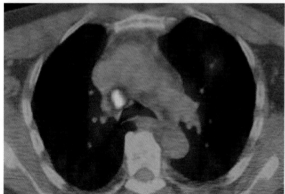

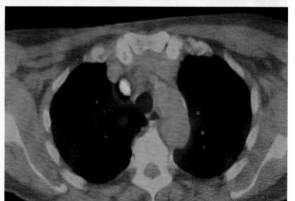

◘ PET findings

increased uptake at the known primary lesions,
omolateral, contralateral and retroclavear nodal
sites of uptake (N3 M0)

Teaching point

Despite the relatively small dimension of the
primary lesion, this case turned out not to be
a candidate for radical surgery.

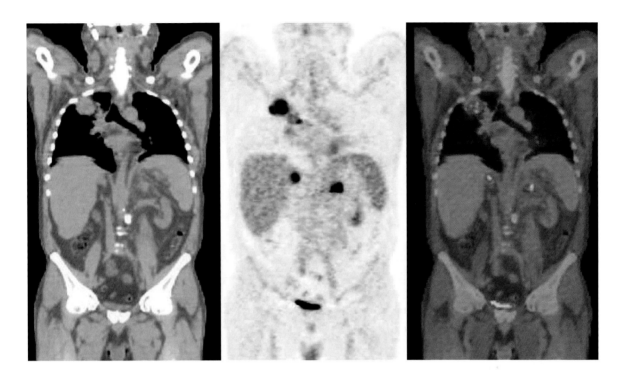

◘ PET findings

increased uptake at the known primary lesions (upper right lung), omolateral, lymph node and both adrenals (N2 M1)

Teaching point

Distant metastases are relatively frequent at presentation of non small cell lung cancer. PET is very useful for some locations, such as adrenal glands, while for the central nervous system CT remains necessary.

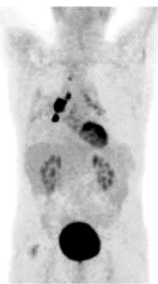

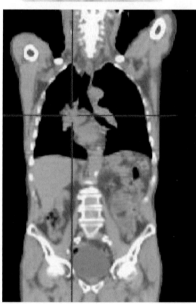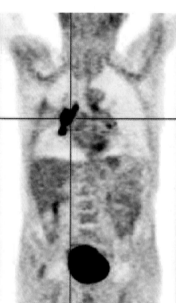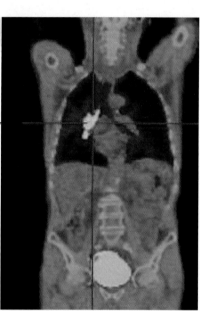

◘ PET findings

increased uptake at the known primary lesions, with other omolateral and contralateral nodal sites of uptake (N3 M0)

Teaching point

Biopsy demonstrated a bronchoalveolar cancer; mediastinoscopy confirmed the nodal staging, thus it was not a candidate for radical surgery. Although the sensitivity of FDG PET can be inferior in bronchoalveolar carcinoma, most cases are FDG avid, and therefore can be staged with PET-CT.

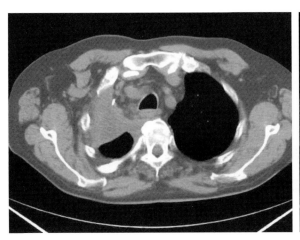 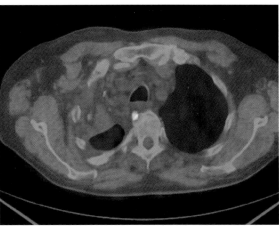

🔲 Previous segmentectomy for right lung adenocarcinoma. Follow-up CT: uncertain finding at the surgical scar.

🔲 **PET findings**

hypermetabolic areas in and around the surgical scar, attributable to local relapse

Teaching point

Studying the tissue metabolism, it is possible to discriminate what is normal, what is fibrosis and what are high metabolic lesions.

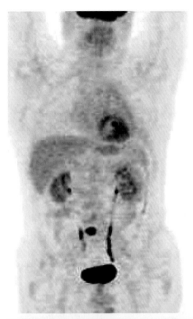

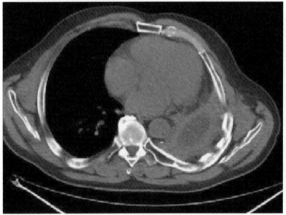
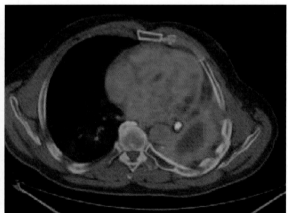

◘ PET findings

hypermetabolic areas near the surgical scar,
attributable to local relapse. Another focal area of
intense uptake consistent with bone metastasis

Case 11   Pneumonectomy for Left Lung Adenocarcinoma. Follow-up CT: Local Relapse

4

Male 72 yo

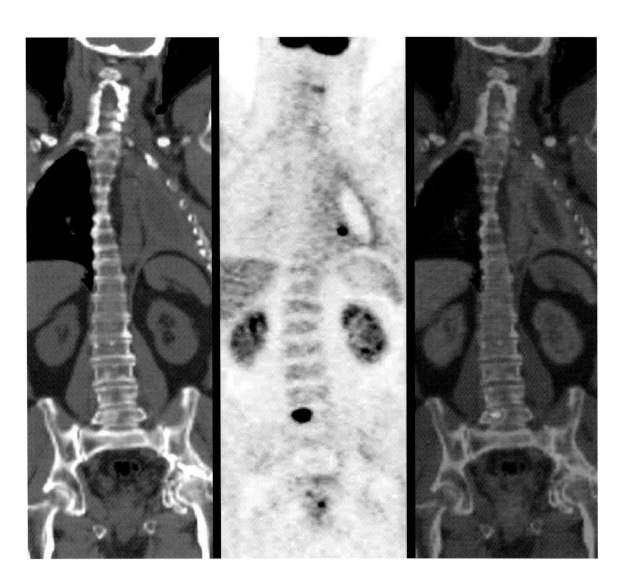

Teaching point

The most appropriate strategy for operated lung cancer is not determined, and CT is most frequently used; in cases of relapse PET is useful to confirm the recurrence and restage the patient.

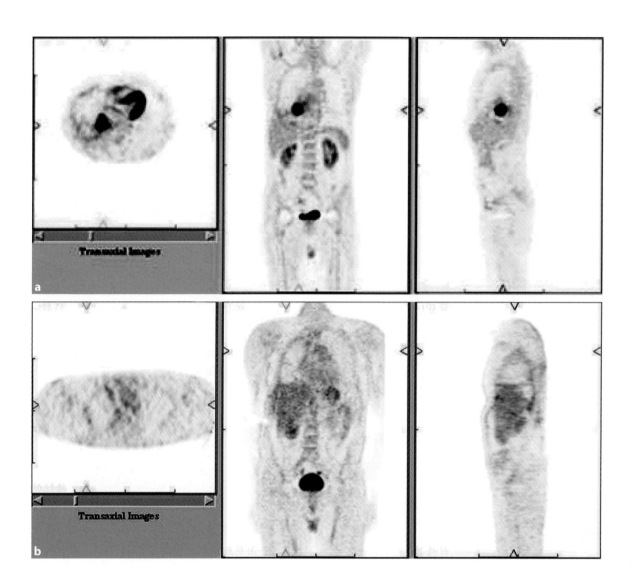

Transaxial Images

a

Transaxial Images

b

▣ PET findings

increased uptake at the known primary lesions before therapy (a), after treatment (b) complete metabolic response (SUV max from 15 to 2)

Teaching point

PET is the most accurate method to evaluate the response to radical radiotherapy or chemotherapy. PET response is significantly associated with survival duration.

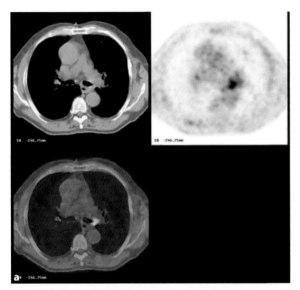

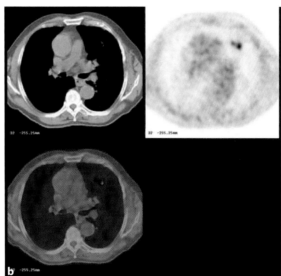

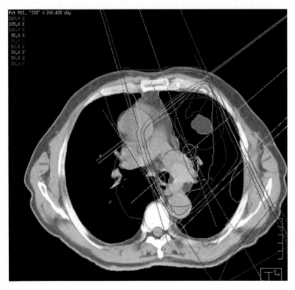

◘ PET findings

PET findings hypermetabolic areas next to the left main bronchus (a) and at parenchyma (b) are used to determine the IMRT plan

Teaching point

Data from PET are useful to plan radiation therapy, especially in lung and neck cancers. Integrated CT and PET data are gaining widespread acceptance to better plan the treatment.

Lymphoma

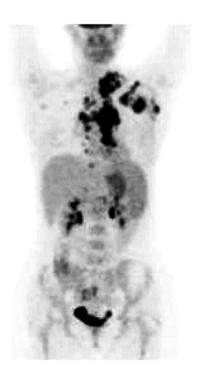

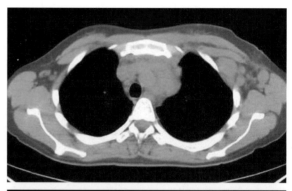

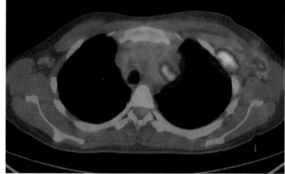

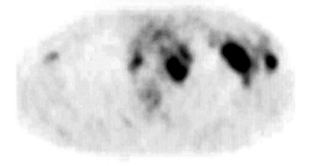

◘ PET findings

several areas of FDG increased uptake in the
mediastinum and at left axillary nodes

Teaching point

PET is highly sensitive in detecting nodal
and extranodal involvement in HD. However,
care has to be paid to some areas where
physiological uptake may occur, like the
stomach and bone marrow (as in this case).

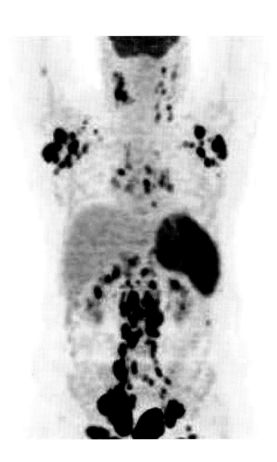

◘ PET findings

many areas of increased uptake in the
laterocervical, axillary, mediastinal, paraaortic,
interaortocaval, iliac and inguinal lymph node.
The spleen is also enlarged and with diffusely
increased uptake, consistent with disease
infiltration

Teaching point

PET is highly sensitive in detecting nodal and
extranodal involvement by most histologic
subtypes of prior lymphoma treatment. Most
common types of lymphoma (e.g., diffuse
large B-cell NHL, follicular NHL, HD) are
routinely FDG avid with a sensitivity and a
specificity that exceeds 90%.

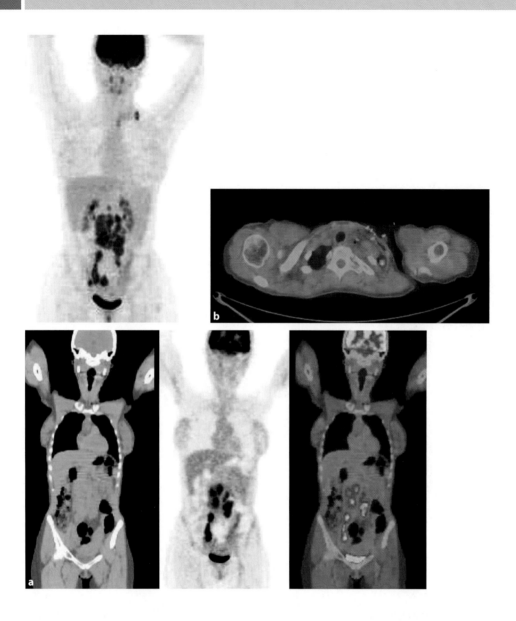

▣ PET findings

many areas of FDG increased uptake in the abdomen (a) and at a left supraclavicular lymph node (b), not known before PET scanning

Teaching point

PET is highly sensitive in lymphoma staging; nonetheless the identification of more involved nodes, as compared to CT, does not necessarily have an impact on patient management. The identification of nodal involvement above the diaphragm in this case modifies the stage and the treatment of the patient.

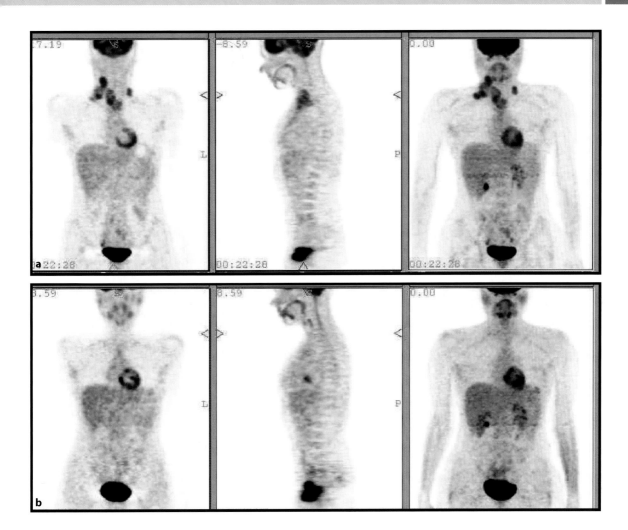

PET findings

staging PET (a) shows some hypermetabolic areas in right laterocervical, bilateral supraclavicular and antero-mediastinal nodes. Post-therapy PET (b): complete response to therapy

Teaching point

PET has been used for early evaluation of HD and NHL during treatment. Early PET scans can be performed after three, two or even one course of chemotherapy, allowing one to discern patients with a good prognosis (early responder) from those with a poor prognosis.

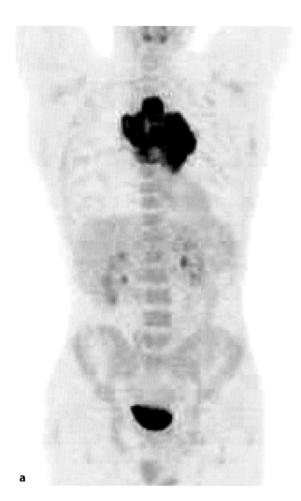

a

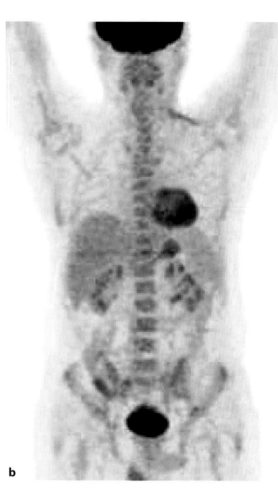

b

◘ PET findings

staging PET (a) shows elevated hypermetabolism of bulky mediastinal mass. Complete remission after chemotherapy + radiotherapy (b)

Teaching point

Despite the complete response, CT imaging shows the bulky mass almost unchanged. Conventional imaging indeed is generally unable to detect the differences between tumor tissue and fibrosis, while PET evaluates metabolism and therefore active residual tumor.

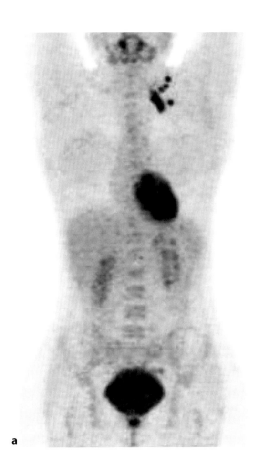

a

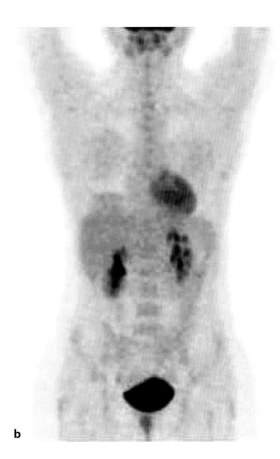

b

◘ PET findings

relapse PET (a) shows active disease at left
supraclavear and antero-mediastinal level.
Complete remission after chemotherapy (b)

Teaching point

PET can demonstrate the response to
treatment after completion of therapy. It
is usually suggested to wait at least four
weeks after chemotherapy completion
and three months after radiotherapy or
radioimmunotherapy completion.

213

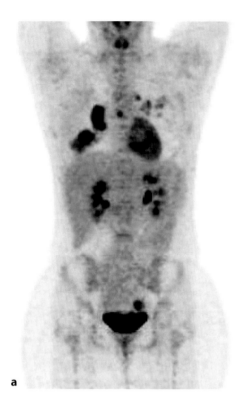
a

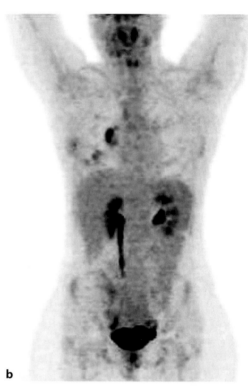
b

◻ PET findings

PET findings relapse PET (a) shows active disease at mediastinal and lung level. Partial remission after chemotherapy (b)

Teaching point

In the first scan (a) a focal area of increased uptake is evident in the left pelvis, consistent with folliculum (physiological finding after ovulation).

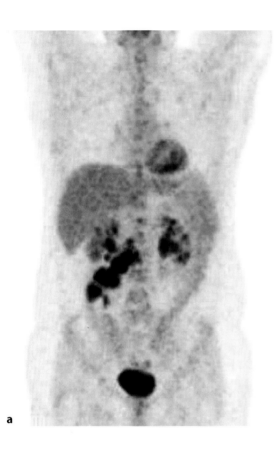

a

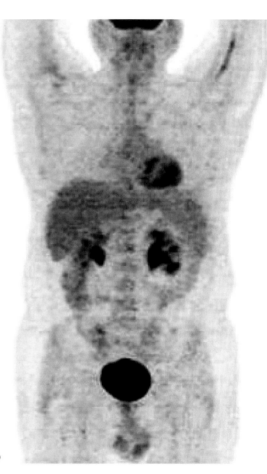

b

▣ PET findings

staging PET (a) shows active disease at bowel level. Complete remission after chemotherapy (b)

Teaching point

PET can also demonstrate the presence and extension of disease in low-grade lymphomas and in challenging localizations (bowel, bone, spleen), even if the accuracy can be lower. In such cases PET can surely be used to evaluate the response to treatment.

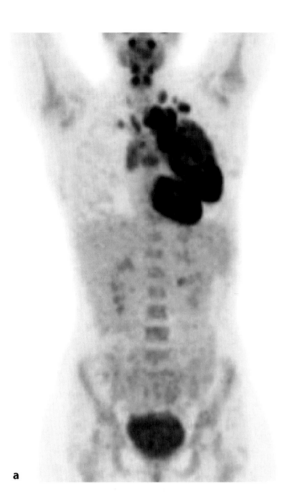

a

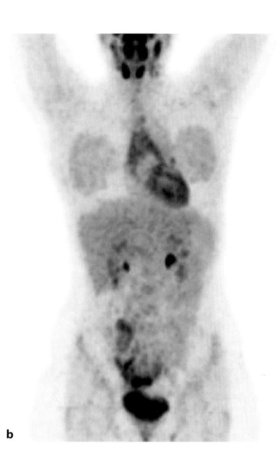

b

◘ PET findings

staging PET (a) shows a large mediastinal mass with involvement of other supradiaphragmatic nodes. Complete response after chemotherapy (b) with evident thymic rebound

Teaching point

In the second scan (b) an increased uptake at anteromediastinal level is evident, with the typical aspect of thymus.

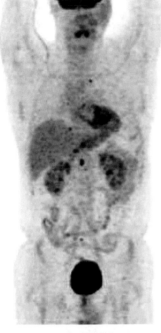

◘ PET findings

several small areas of increased uptake at lymph nodes (not enlarged at CT), consistent with residual disease

Teaching point

PET can demonstrate the presence of residual disease more accurately than CT findings.

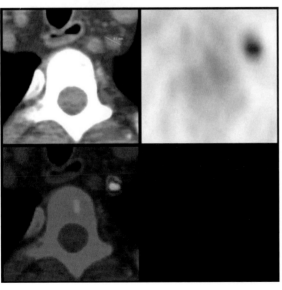

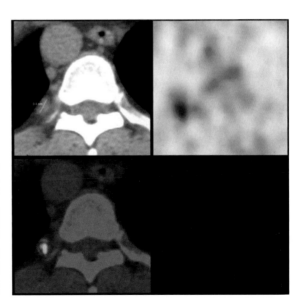

4

Case 11   **NHL in Complete Remission. After Chemotherapy**

Female 45 yo

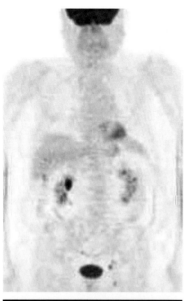

◘ NHL in complete remission after chemotherapy. Follow-up scan. Primitive sites of disease: spleen and right inguinal lymph nodes.

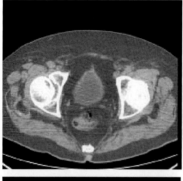

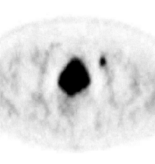

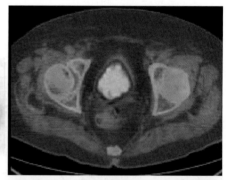

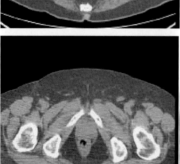

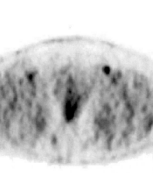

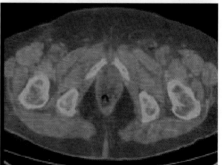

◘ PET findings

two hypermetabolic inguinal left lymph nodes, consistent with relapse (confirmed at biopsy)

Teaching point

In aggressive NHL patients and high-risk HD, the use of PET may be suggested during follow-up, allowing an earlier detection of relapse (before clinical symptoms) and therefore an earlier treatment.

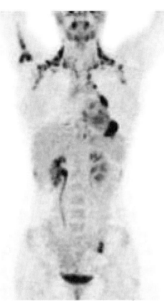

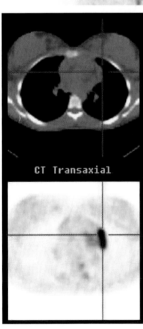

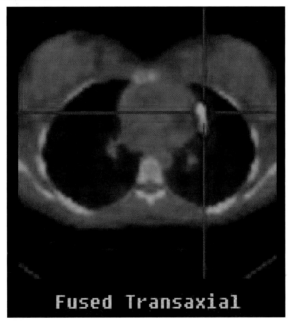

CT Transaxial

Fused Transaxial

◘ PET findings

several areas of FDG increased uptake in the mediastinum, bilateral supraclavicular (brown fat), paracardiac, right homerus and left iliac wing (recurrence)

Teaching point

In the presence of contemporary relapse and brown fat, the degree of uptake has limited value to discriminate the finding. PET-CT is necessary to identify the sites of relapse.

Melanoma

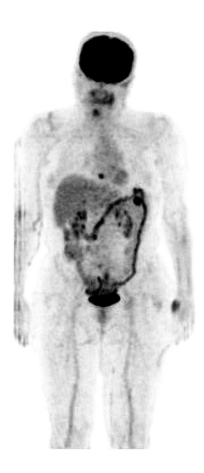

PET findings

two hypermetabolic areas at bone and spleen, respectively

Teaching point

Melanoma of the skin may spread either locally or regionally and to distant sites through predictable or unpredictable metastatic pathways. For this reason it is important to acquire a real whole body scan. In this case is also evident the increased uptake in the bowel, especially in the distal colon, not attributable to oncological origin but simply to inflammatory and irritative causes.

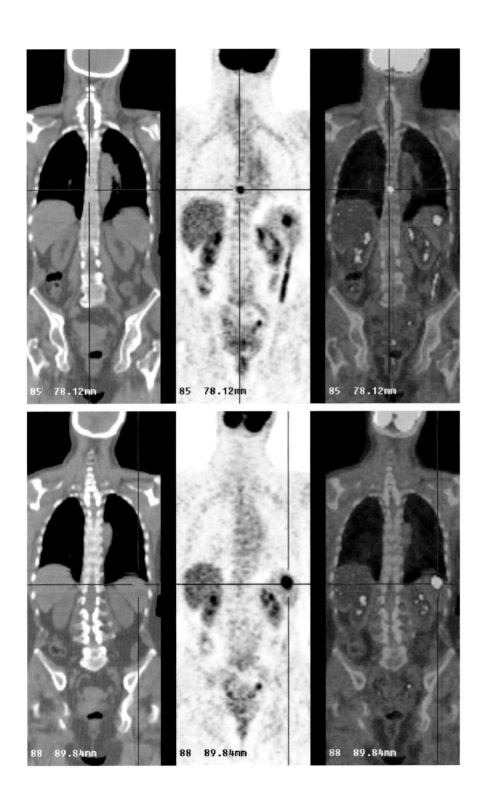

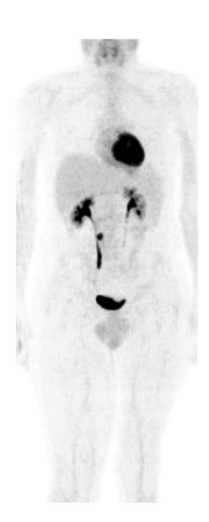

◘ PET findings

hypermetabolism of one abdominal lymph node
refers to metastasis

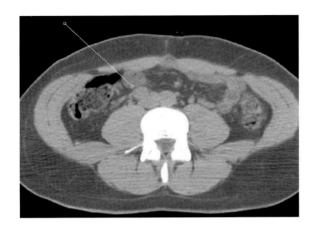

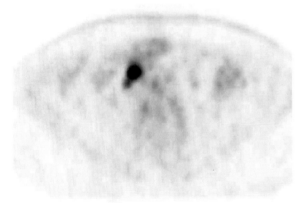

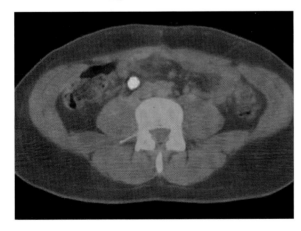

Teaching point

Staging FDG-PET scanning did not impact the care of patients with early-stage melanoma. On the other hand cumulative data suggest that FDG-PET is the modality of choice for:

- individuals with a high risk for distant metastases based on the extent of locoregional disease
- patients with findings that are suspicious for distant metastases
- individuals with known distant tumor deposits who still stand to benefit from customized therapies if new lesions are discovered or treated lesions regress
- patients at high risk for systemic relapse who are considering aggressive medical therapy.

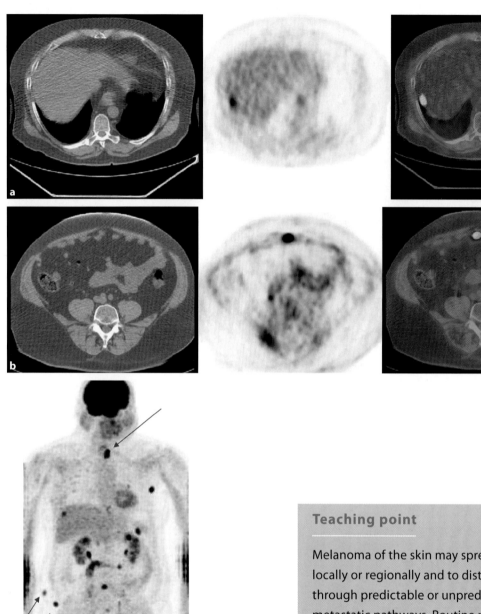

▣ PET findings

hypermetabolic areas at the soft tissue of paravertebral region, loin and gluteus (red arrows on MIP), axillary and abdominal lymph nodes (b) and liver (a)

Teaching point

Melanoma of the skin may spread either locally or regionally and to distant sites through predictable or unpredictable metastatic pathways. Routine protocols based on clinical examinations and traditional radiologic evaluations are not cost-effective for the detection of systemic disease. In the last decade, nuclear medicine techniques, such as lymphoscintigraphy-directed lymphatic mapping with sentinel lymphadenectomy and PET, have played key roles in nodal and distant staging of melanoma.

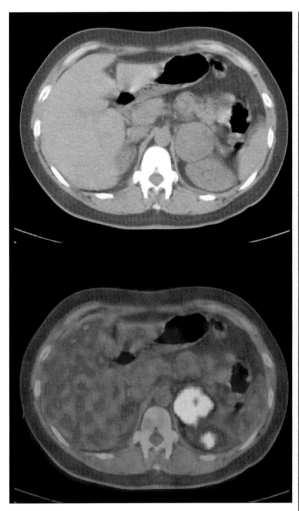

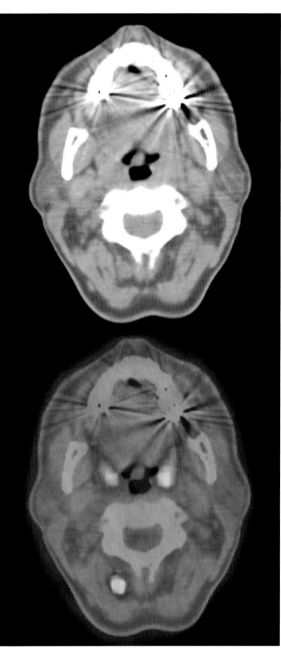

227

PET findings

increased uptake at left adrenal mass and demonstration of uptake at a nucal lymph node

Teaching point

PET is useful for re-staging melanoma patient with suspected recurrence.

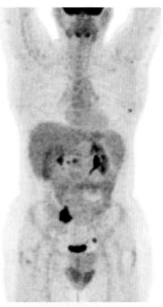

◑ PET findings

several hypermetabolic areas at abdominal and pelvic lymph nodes and at chest soft tissue

Teaching point

The localization of recurrence sites of melanoma may be difficult, and CT images are almost necessary to properly identify the lesions.

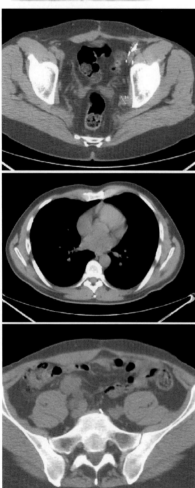

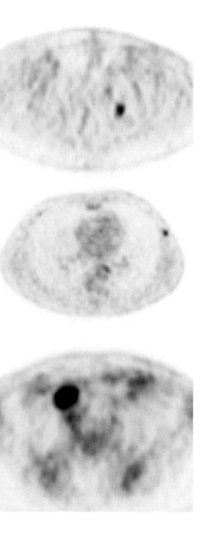

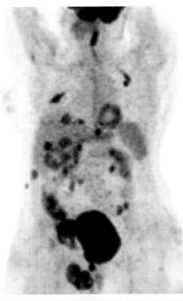

▣ PET findings

several areas of increased uptake at local level, bones, lung and liver

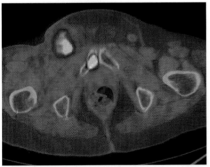
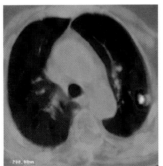
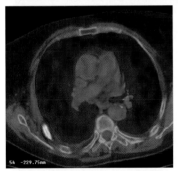
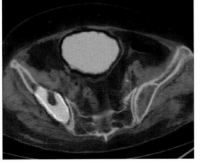
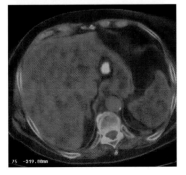

Teaching point

While staging FDG-PET scanning is not routinely used in melanoma patients, restaging in advanced disease can be usefully applied.

Mesothelioma

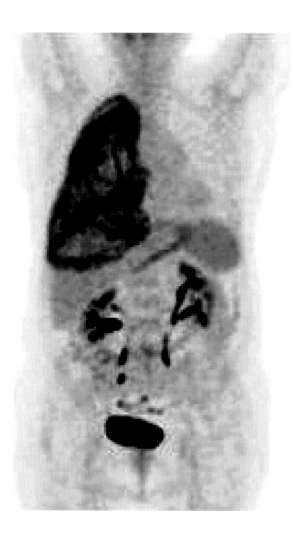

◧ PET findings

diffuse and increased FDG uptake at all the right pleura. No other site of pathologic uptake

Teaching point

PET-CT seems to be a valuable tool in staging of Malignant Pleural Mesothelioma (MPM) compared to CT alone. In many cases these differences are clinically relevant and have therapeutic consequences.

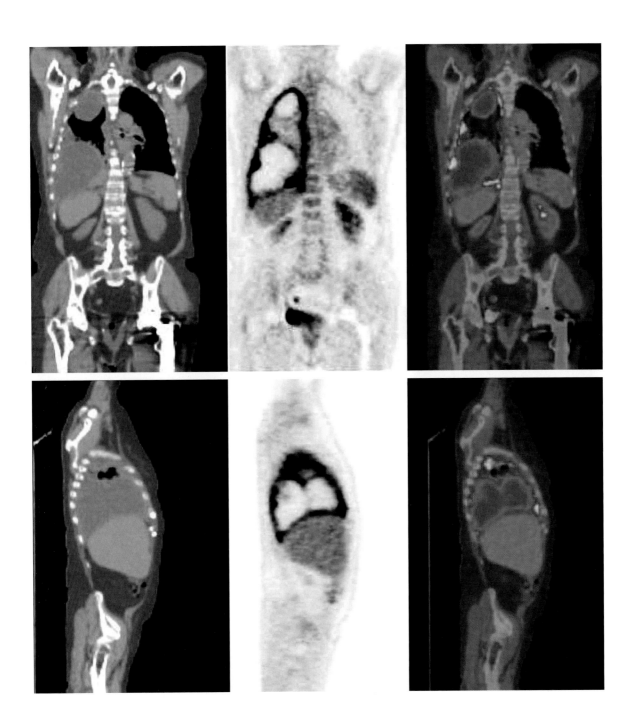

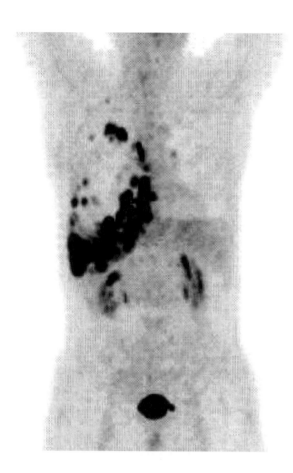

◘ PET findings

many confluent areas of intense FDG uptake at the right pleura. A small nodule is also affecting the contralateral pleura

Teaching point

In cases of surgical approach, PET is important to evaluate the extent of the disease.

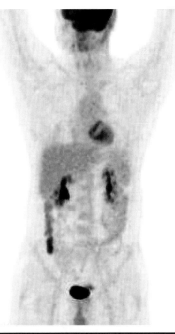

◘ PET findings

non pathologic uptake of FDG. Complete metabolic response to therapy

Teaching point

PET is useful in the evaluation of MPM, giving additional data that can clarify doubtful CT findings, especially regarding lymph node involvement, pleural thickening after therapy and distant site of metastasis.

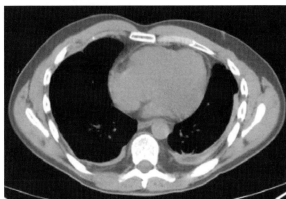

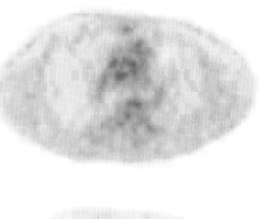

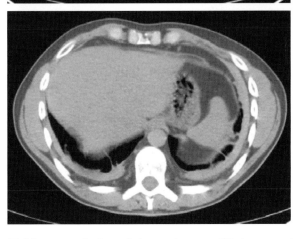

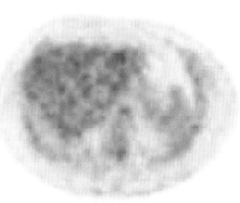

◘ After completion of chemotherapy, CT shows a pleural thickening of uncertain significance.

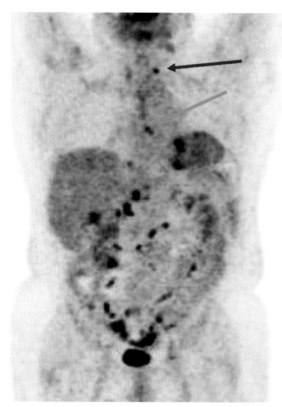

◘ PET findings

multiple small hypermetabolic peritoneal nodules refers to known disease. Thyroid nodule (red arrow) and post-surgical changes at the sternum (green arrow) are visible

Teaching point

There is no literature on the value of staging peritoneal mesothelioma by PET. Nevertheless it seems to be a useful tool due to its intrinsic capacity to study changes in metabolic behavior. On the other hand, different lesions due to oncological and non oncological reasons can show a similar degree of FDG uptake.

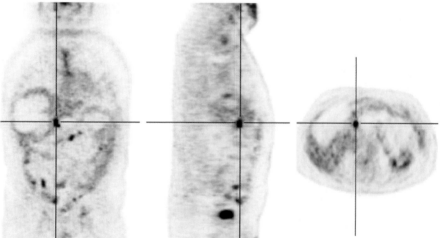

◘ Peritoneal mesothelioma PET staging. Left thyroid lobe affected by nodules. 6 years ago sternotomy for cardiosurgery intervention.

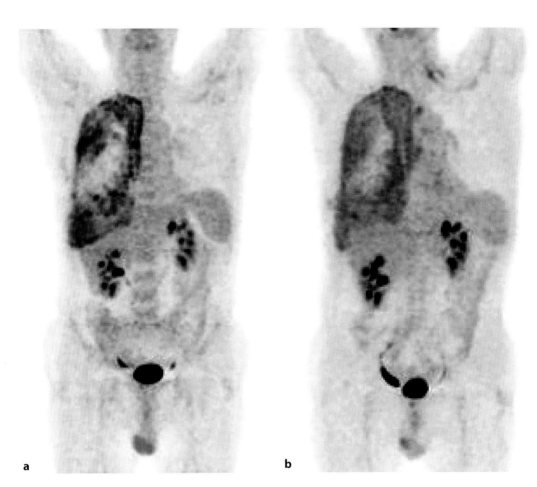

a   b

◘ Pleural mesothelioma: staging (a,c) and post-therapy after 3 months (b,d).

◘ PET findings

at staging (a,c), right pleura is diffusely hypermetabolic (SUVmax = 10). After chemotherapy (b,d) PET shows a decrease of glucose uptake (SUVmax = 5.4), but the appearance of two new hypermetabolic mediastinal adenopathies (red arrow)

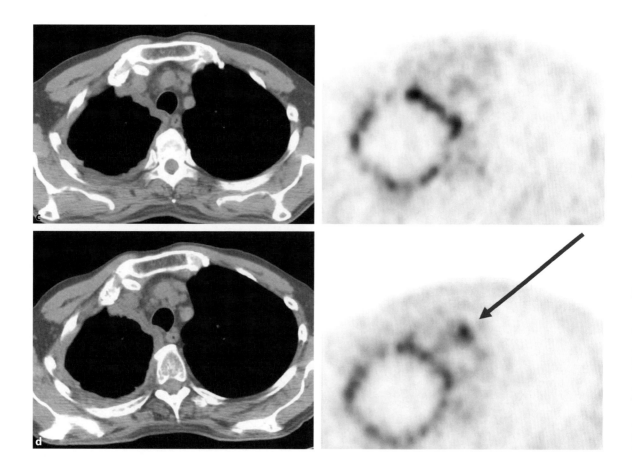

Teaching point

PET scan in malignant pleural mesothelioma allows a correct post-therapy restaging (metabolism reduction of the primary tumor). Furthermore, in this case the presence of mediastinal lymph nodes modifies TNM classification (N2).

Other

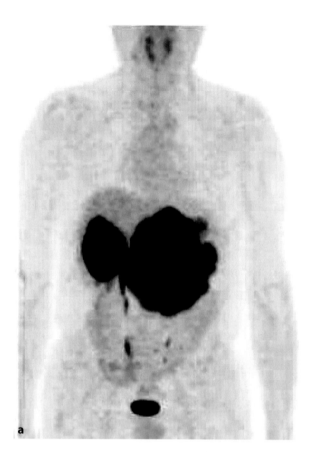

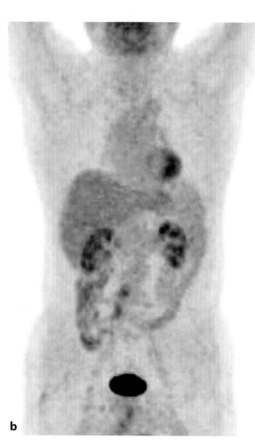

PET findings

Staging PET (a) shows the huge hypermetabolic lesion; after therapy PET shows an impressive complete metabolic response (b)

Teaching point

FDG-PET can be used to stage GIST and evaluate the response to treatment.

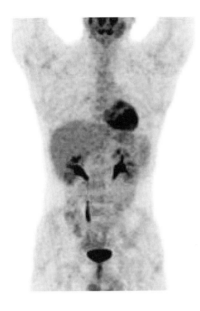

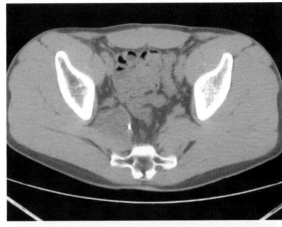

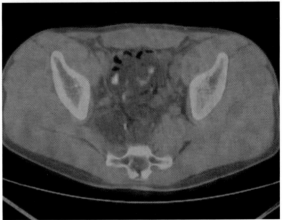

◘ PET findings

increased uptake at the pelvic mass

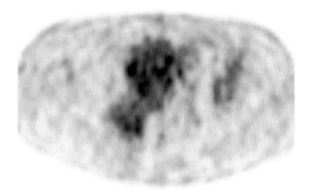

4

Case 3   **Recent Surgery for Cholangiocarcinoma. Suspected Liver Recurrence**

Female 68 yo

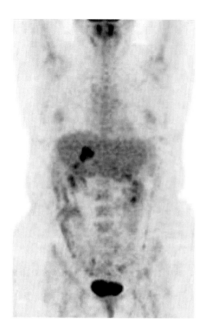

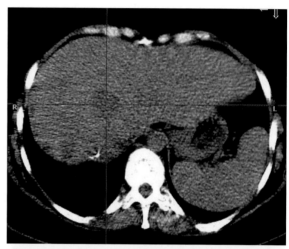

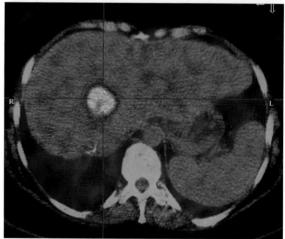

◘ PET findings

large hypermetabolic lesion at hepatic level

Teaching point

PET can be usefully employed to clarify uncertain findings, as well as to evaluate the extent of suspected relapse.

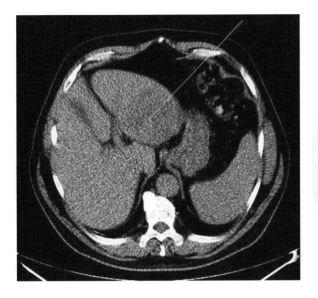

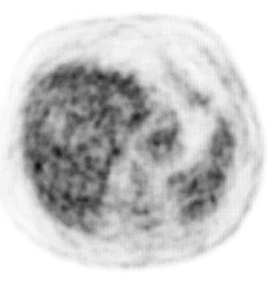

▣ PET findings

lack of uptake at the mass

Teaching point

Hepatocellular carcinoma can be FDG negative. Therefore, FDG PET has a limited role to evaluate this disease.

4

Case 5   Previous Surgery for Bladder Cancer. Suspected Recurrence

Male 59 yo

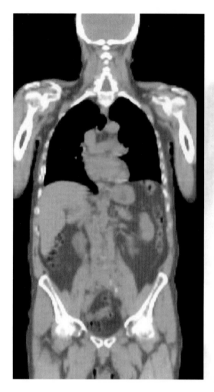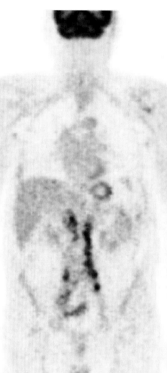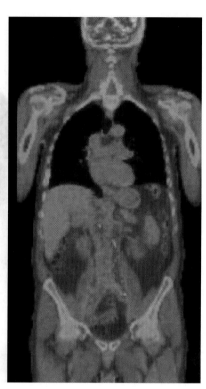

▣ PET findings

increased uptake at abdominal lymph nodes

Teaching point

PET can be usefully employed to evaluate the extent of relapse in bladder cancer.

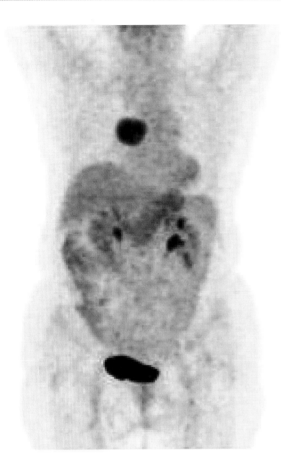

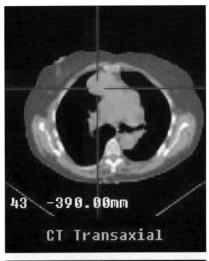

CT Transaxial

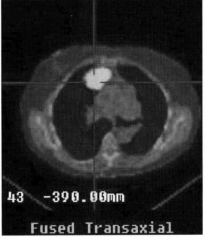

Fused Transaxial

▣ PET findings

large hypermetabolic lesion at mediastinum; biopsy revealed a thymoma, subsequently surgically removed

Teaching point

FDG PET can provide information about the possible malignant nature of the lesion, but a final pathologic diagnosis can be made only by biopsy.

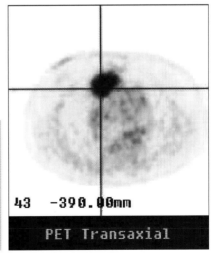

PET Transaxial

245

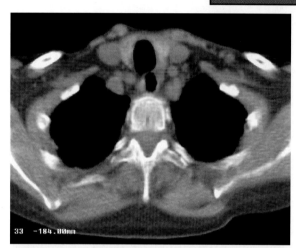

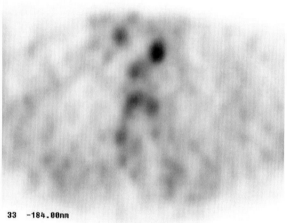

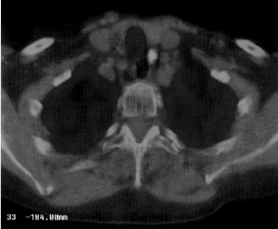

◻ 11C-METH

◻ Patient affected by secondary hyperparathyroidism due to renal failure on chronic haemodialysis. Dual-phase 99mTc-sestamibi imaging is negative.

◻ 11C methionine PET findings

one hypermetabolic area behind the left lobe of the thyroid refers to one hyperfunctioned parathyroid

Teaching point

The mechanisms of accumulation of methionine by parathyroid tissues are transmembrane amino acid transport, protein synthesis and methionine donor transmethylation. Studies in hyperparathyroidism have demonstrated that accumulation of 11C-methionine is correlated with serum parathyroid hormone and calcium levels. 11C-methionine PET/CT may be used to identify hyperfunctioning parathyroid glands in non-primary hyperparathyroidism when conventional 99 mTc-sestamibi imaging is non-localizing.

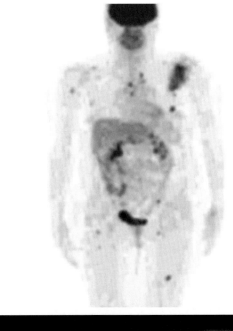

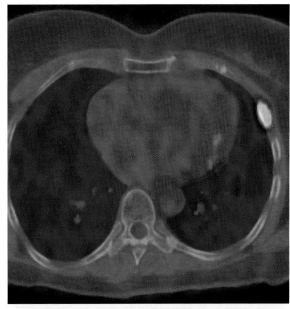

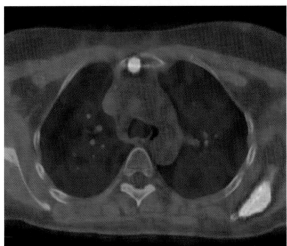

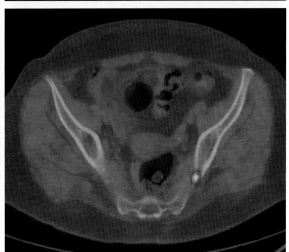

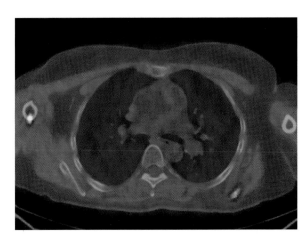

◘ PET findings

multiple hypermetabolic lesions of the homerus, scapule, rib, pelvis, sternum and femur

Teaching point

Currently, conventional radiographic skeletal surveys, magnetic resonance imaging, and F-18 FDG PET/CT examinations are the most useful instruments for staging myeloma.

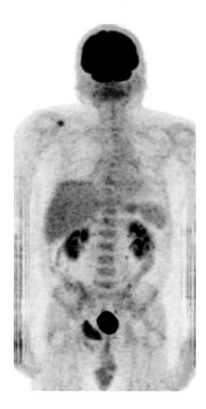

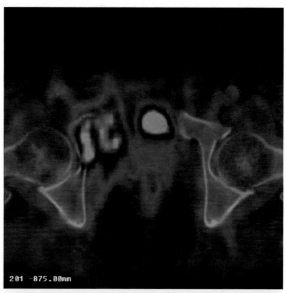

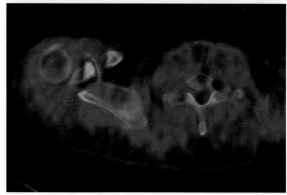

■ PET findings

increased uptake at pelvic known lesion; evidence
of another lesion at right scapulae

Teaching point

At disease presentation, it is particularly
important to identify all active lesions, as
treatment of multiple myeloma may be
different in cases of solitary lesions. In these
infrequent cases PET should be performed
in order to rule out the presence of other
localizations.

Ovarian Cancer

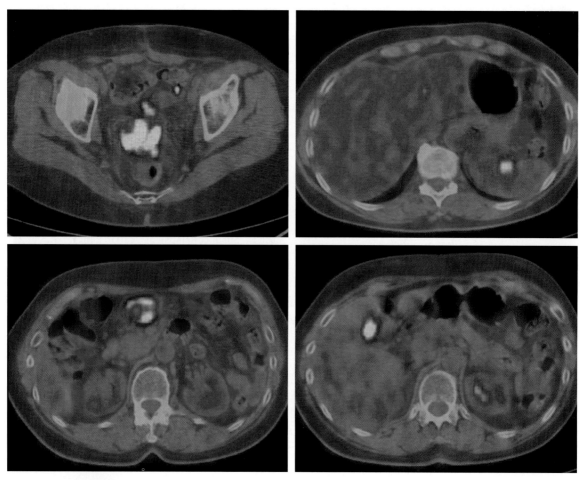

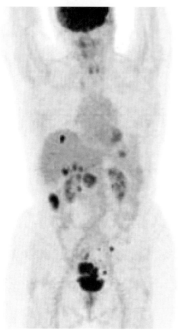

PET findings

staging PET shows primary lesion and disease
diffusion to several lymph nodes

Teaching point

At presentation, most women have stage III
or stage IV disease. The overall 5-year survival
rate is therefore only between 25% and 40%.
Metastasis in ovarian cancer can occur by
seeding or shedding into the abdominal
cavity involving the layer of omentum and
the capsule of the liver (Stage III).

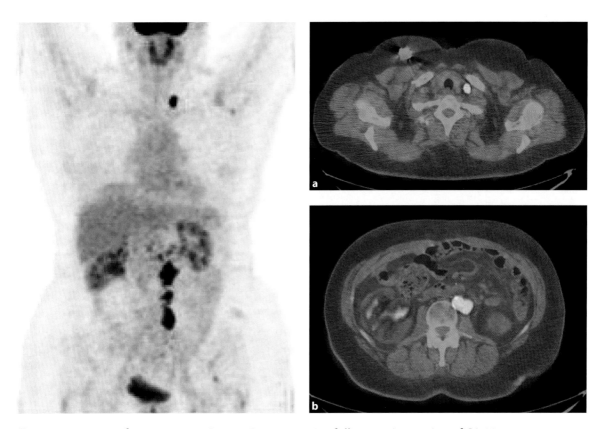

🔲 Previous surgery for ovarian carcinoma. Post-operative follow-up. Increasing of CA 125.

🔲 PET findings

disease diffusion to left supraclavear adenopathy
(a) and lombo-aortic lymph nodes (b)

Teaching point

Epithelial ovarian cancer is the leading
cause of death from gynecological cancer in
Western countries. Approximately 20–30%
of patients with early-stage disease and
50–75% of those with advanced disease who
obtain a complete response will ultimately
develop recurrent disease.

4

Case 3   **Previous Surgery for Ovarian Carcinoma. Post-operative Follow-up**

Female 38 yo

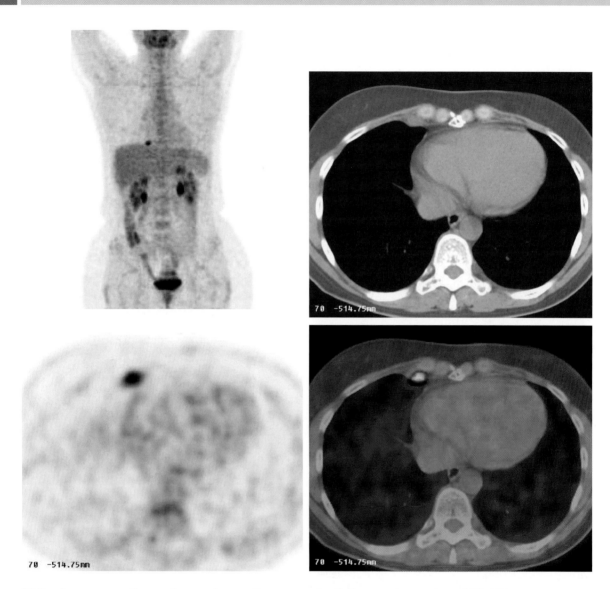

◻ Previous surgery for ovarian carcinoma. Post-operative follow-up. Increasing of CA 125.

◻ PET findings

small area of increased uptake, consistent with pleural lesion

Teaching point

Suspect relapse is likely the most frequent reason for performing a PET in patients with ovarian cancer. FDG PET has a sensitivity of about 90% and a specificity of about 85% for the detection of recurrent disease.

Case 4   **Previous Surgery (BIA) for Ovarian Carcinoma. Post-operative Follow-up**

Female 63 yo

4

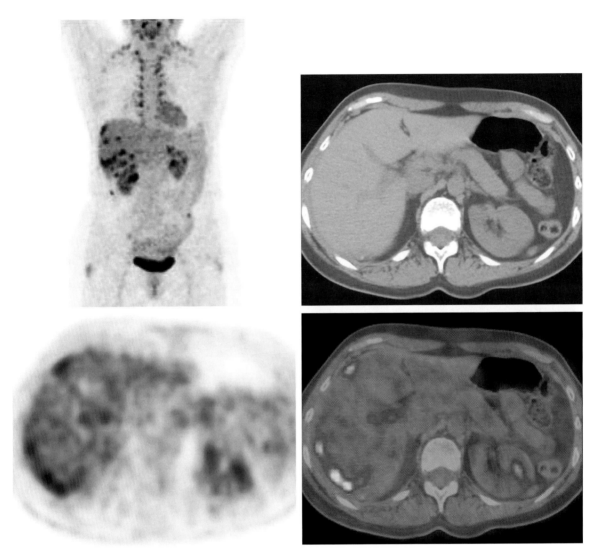

🔲 Previous surgery (BIA) for ovarian carcinoma. Post-operative follow-up. Increasing of CA 125.

🔲 PET findings

shows disease diffusion to liver capsule

Teaching point

Carcinosis is a relatively frequent form of ovarian cancer spread, making early diagnosis challenging for any given imaging procedure. PET usually detects early carcinomatosis as liver capsule diffusion. The patient has also an evident visualization of brown fat.

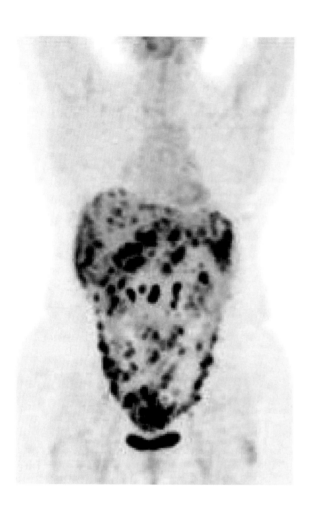

◘ PET findings

increased uptake to omentum, refers to peritoneal carcinosis

Teaching point

Since the original description of the "seed and soil" hypothesis by Paget, the importance of a specific host environment has been recognized as a key factor in the development of tumor metastasis. The peritoneal cytokine, adhesion molecule and growth factor environment largely determine the growth of cancerous implants on the peritoneal mesothelium.

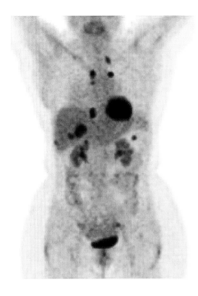

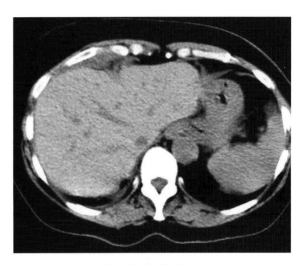

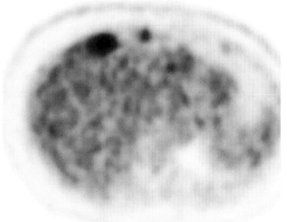

◘ Patient operated for ovarian cancer, increased markers, negative US and abdominal CT.

◘ PET findings

several areas of focal FDG uptake below and above the diaphragm, at lymph nodes and likely carcinosis nodes

Teaching point

CT can be negative due to lack of exploration (thorax CT is not frequently performed in ovarian cancer patients) but also due to lesions overlooking.

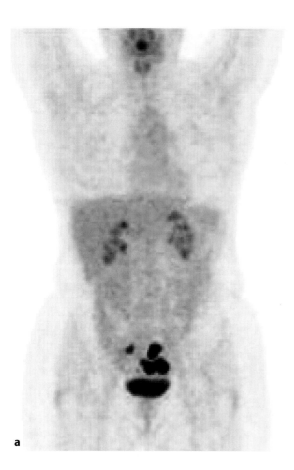

a

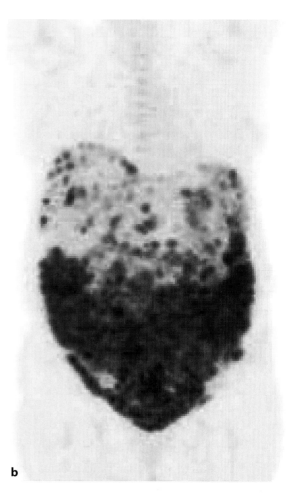

b

◘ PET findings

FDG increased uptake in peritoneal carcinosis.
Case (a) very faint increase of tracer uptake; case
(b) diffuse massive increase

Teaching point

Identification of peritoneal carcinosis is
challenging for every imaging method, in
particular at early diffusion. FDG PET can
easily be interpreted in advanced disease,
while initial diagnosis is difficult.

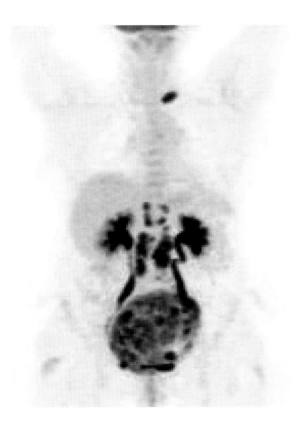

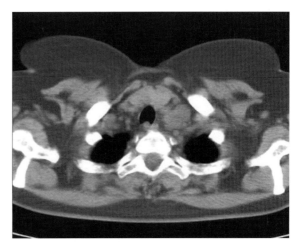

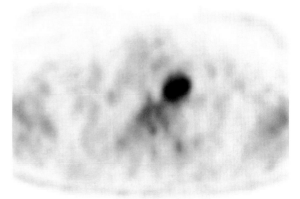

◘ PET findings

large mass and increased uptake at several
abdominal lymph nodes; also one retroclavear
node is involved

Teaching point

Ovarian cancer usually diffuses to local
lymph nodes and to the peritoneal cavity;
supra diaphragmatic spread is regarded as
distant metastases. However, in advanced
disease the diffusion to left supraclavear
nodes can be observed with FDG PET.

Pancreas

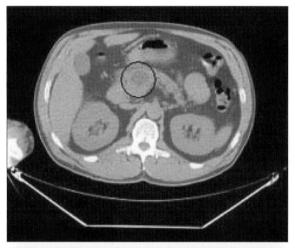

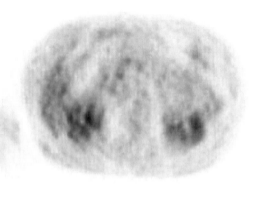

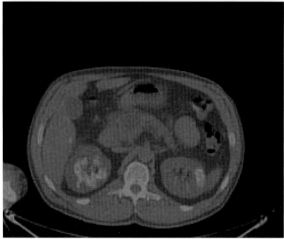

◘ PET findings

no pathologic uptake at the cystic lesion: at
follow-up no malignancy

Teaching point

Both chronic pancreatitis and pancreatic
cancer may present as a pancreatic mass.
Differentiation of these disease entities is
fundamental because of the tremendously
different management, treatment and
prognostic implications. Sensitivity and
specificity of FDG-PET for the diagnosis
of malignancy is about 90% and 85%
respectively, significantly superior to CT.

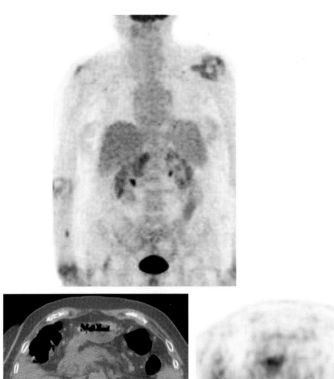

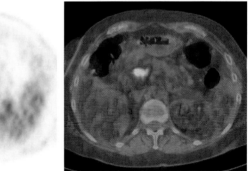

◘ Patient with epigastric pain and increased Ca 19-9. CT scan shows a pancreatic mass suspected for tumor.

◘ **FDG findings:**

hypermetabolic lesion at pancreatic head refers to malignancy. Note several areas of increased uptake due to arthrosis

Teaching point

The functional imaging approach of nuclear medicine offers important information for the characterization of suspected lesions.

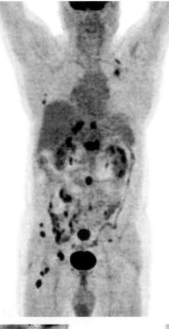

◘ PET findings

two hypermetabolic lesions of the right lung, with several bones and lymph node lesions

> **Teaching point**
>
> In patients suspected of pancreatic cancer relapse, FDG-PET reliably detected local recurrences, whereas CT is more sensitive for the detection of hepatic metastases. Furthermore, PET proved to be advantageous for the detection of nonlocoregional and extra-abdominal recurrences.

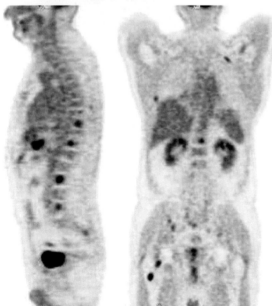
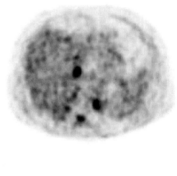

◘ Subtotal pancreasectomy for adenocarcinoma and subsequent chemotherapy with complete remission. Five years later increase of CA 19.9. CT scan shows one small (1 cm) area at inferior lobe of right lung, reported as indeterminate

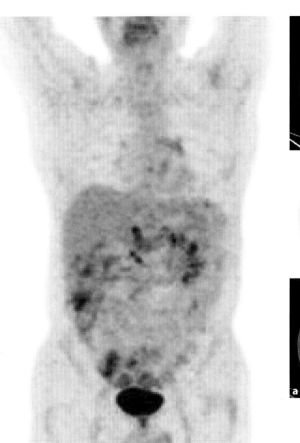

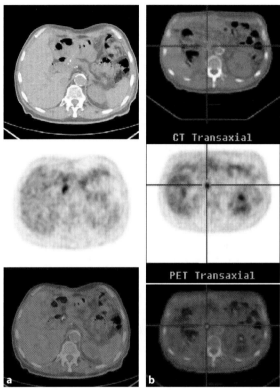

■ Previous duodenocefalopancreasectomy for biliopancreatic tumor; ten years before right nefrectomy for renal adenocarcinoma.
CT scan during follow-up shows peripancreatic and periduodenal lymph node enlargement, suspected for metastasis.

263

■ **FDG findings**

hypermetabolic pancreatic small area in surgical site (a) and one hypermetabolic interaortocaval lymph node (b), both refer to relapse

Teaching point

Anatomical changing after surgical intervention make local relapse assessment difficult, due to the presence of scars. Metabolic imaging provides the ability to evaluate the real situation inside the tissue.

Prostate

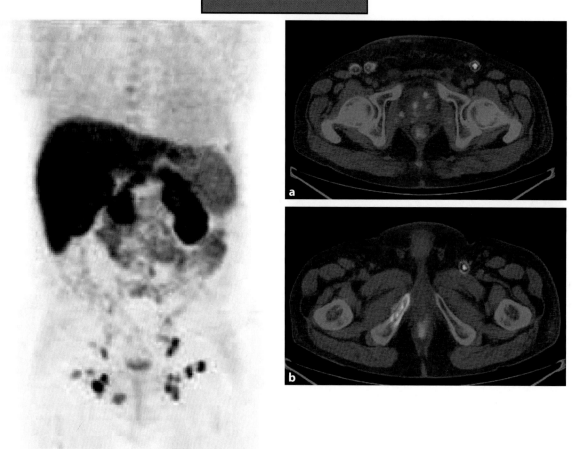

^{11}C-CHOL

☐ Previous radiation therapy for prostate cancer (three years before); recent increase of PSA (24 ng/mL). Androgen therapy on course.

☐ 11C choline PET findings

several hypermetabolic lesions at lymph nodes (a) and bones (b)

Teaching point

Choline PET can usefully be employed to detect recurrence of prostate cancer, since it is able to demonstrate relapse either local, nodal or distant.

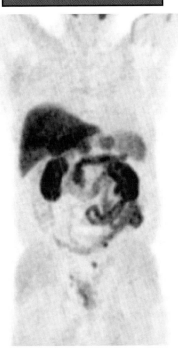

¹¹C-CHOL

◘ 11C choline PET findings

one hypermetabolic lesion in the prostatic gland and two hypermetabolic left iliac lymph nodes. The definitive pathological staging was T2a and 2/18 positive lymph nodes

Teaching point

Although PET imaging has a wide field of view (fundamental for distant metastasis assessing), choline PET can understage prostate cancer, especially if a nerve-sparing RP is considered.

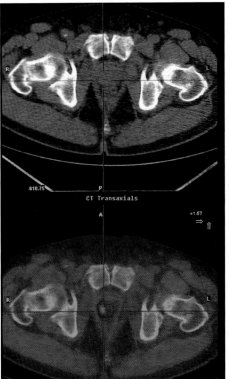

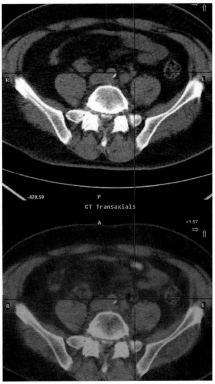

¹¹C-CHOL

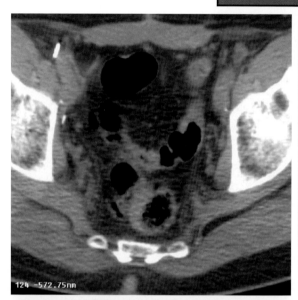

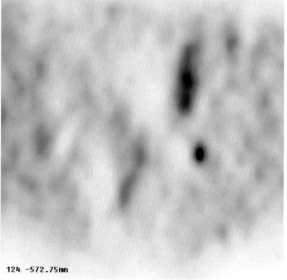

◘ Prostatectomy + radiotherapy three years before. After one year PSA increasing (from 1.18 to 1.57 in last two months). No hormonal therapy. TRUS and biopsy were negative

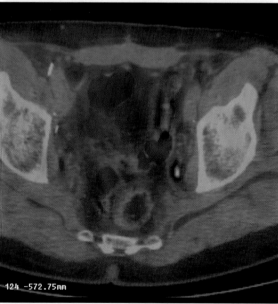

◘ 11C choline PET findings

one hypermetabolic left iliac lymph node

Teaching point

In the majority of cases of prostate cancer recurrence is suspected with the increasing of PSA levels.

Soft-Tissue Tumors

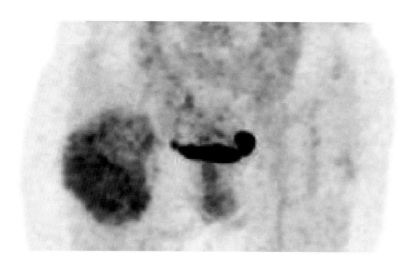

◘ FDG PET-CT shows increased uptake at thigh
mass (SUV = 7.2)

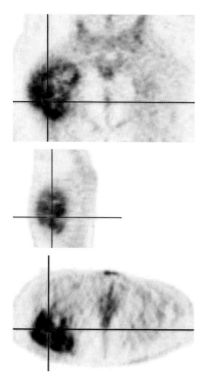

Teaching point

FDG PET has a prognostic significance in
patients with resectable soft tissue sarcoma.
In this case the expected five-year survival,
despite the lack of metastases, is < 20%.

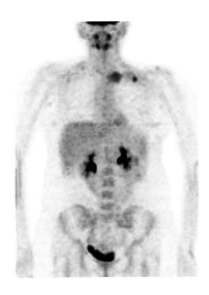

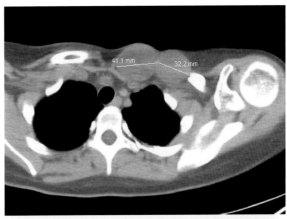

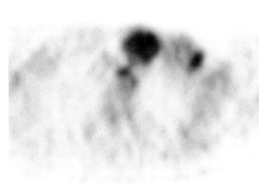

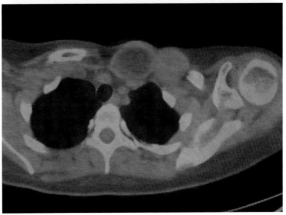

◻ FDG PET-CT shows a faint increase of uptake at both masses

Teaching point

FDG PET has a good but excellent sensitivity (50–95%) to diagnose malignant soft tissue lesions.

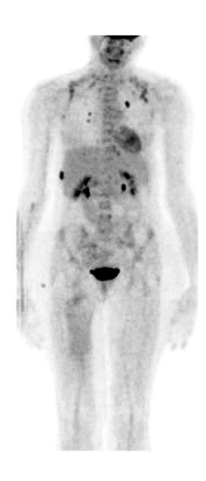

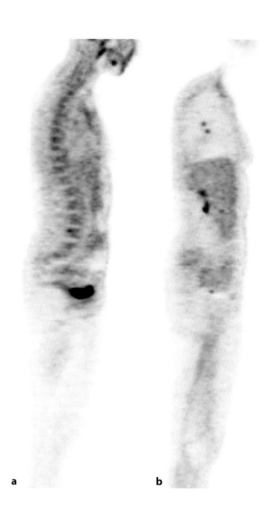

a   b

▣ FDG PET-CT shows other sites of secondary lesions at L4 (a) and two right lung nodules (b)

Teaching point

FDG PET has higher sensitivity to detect distant metastasis as compared to CT and MRI.

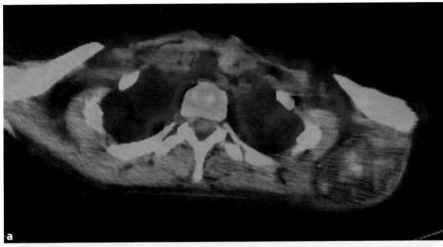

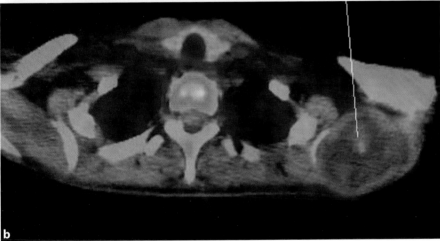

◘ PET findings

increased FDG uptake at presentation (a). Mild decrease of uptake (SUV decrease = – 35%) after therapy completion, partial response (b)

Teaching point

PET is useful for evaluating the response to treatment and provides prognostic information, such as SUV reduction < 40% represent a high risk of recurrence.

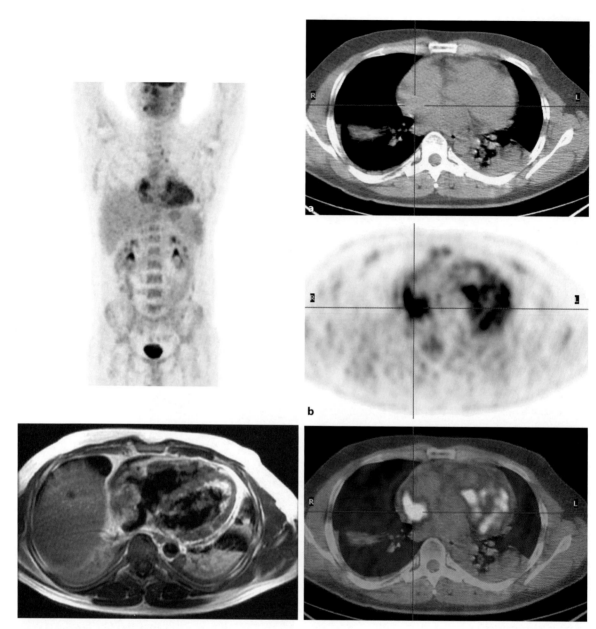

🔲 Cardiac tamponade; MR showed one right atrial mass with irregular contrast enhancement and pericardial infiltration (a)

🔲 **FDG-PET findings**

atrial lesion demonstrates increased glucose uptake (SUVmax 8.7)

Teaching point

In rare cases such as atrial lesions, in which biopsy is difficult if not impossible, metabolic evaluation with PET could discern malign vs. benign tumor.

Case 6   **Sarcoma of Soft Tissue Around the Right Clavicle. Staging PET**

Female 36 yo

4

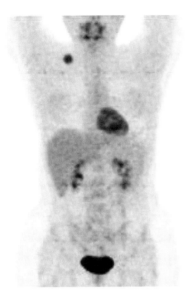

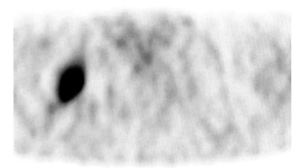

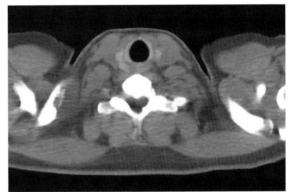

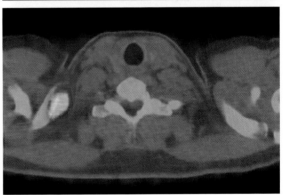

◘ PET findings

area of FDG increased uptake at the known
clavicular lesion (SUVmax = 7.1)

Teaching point

PET-CT provides the correct staging in a high
percentage of patients (about 90%).

Testicular Cancer

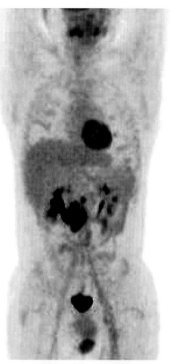

PET findings

intense uptake at the abdominal mass, no other sites of pathologic uptake

Teaching point

In presence of suspected finding at CT, the utility of PET is due to its capability in restaging.

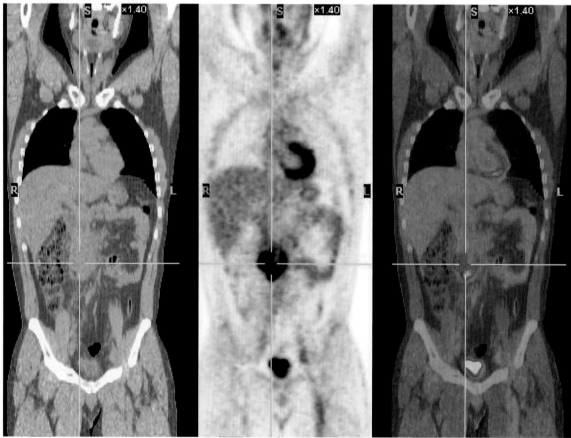

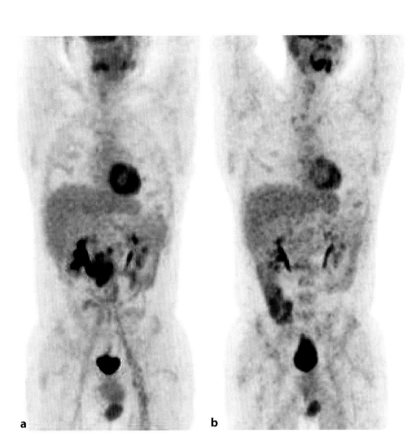

a   b

PET findings

before chemotherapy, intense uptake at the abdominal mass (a), and after treatment complete metabolic response (b)

Teaching point

PET can be usefully employed to evaluate response to therapy. In the second scan a non-focal uptake at the bowel is evident, more intense in the caecal area, not attibutable to pathological cause.

4

Case 3   **Testicular Cancer. Follow-up After Surgery.and Chemotherapy**

Male 44 yo

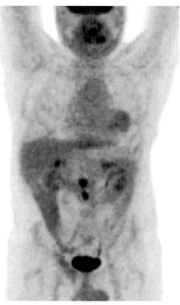

◼ PET findings

two hypermetabolic abdominal adenopathy

Teaching point

Though PET identified some patients with disease not detected by computed tomography scan, in patients at low risk of relapse the rate of recurrent disease among PET negative remains high.

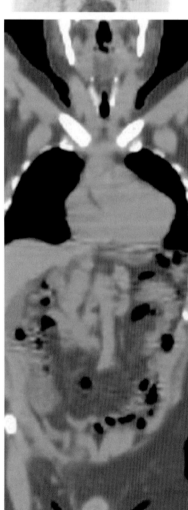

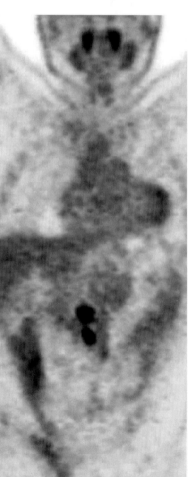

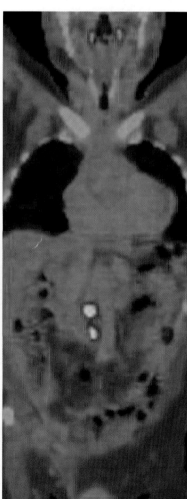

Thyroid

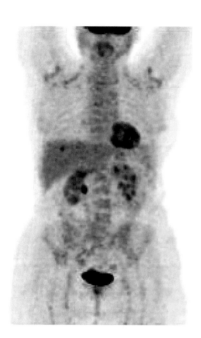

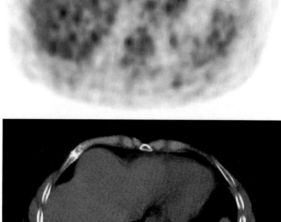

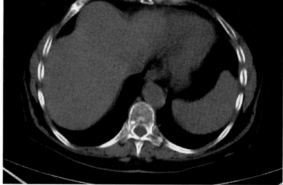

▣ PET findings

focal FDG increased uptake at VII right rib

Teaching point

FDG PET is useful in assessing recurrent or metastatic lesions in patients with increased thyroglobulin and 131 I scan-negative.

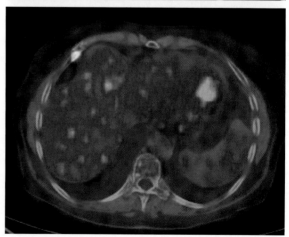

▣ Patient treated with surgery and radioiodine therapy. Thyreoglobuline increase with negative radioiodine whole body scan.

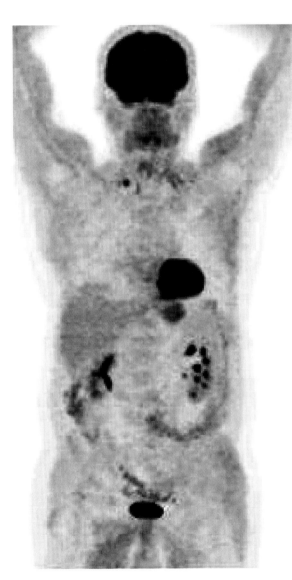

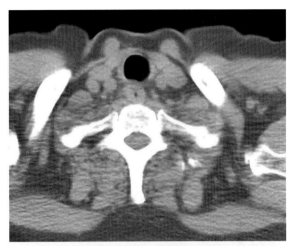

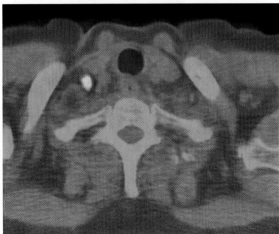

◘ Thyroid carcinoma after surgery. Tg increasing with negative radioiodine whole body scan.

◘ PET findings

focal FDG increased uptake at lymph node

Teaching point

FDG PET is useful in assessing recurrent disease in patients with increased thyroglobulin and 131 I scan-negative.

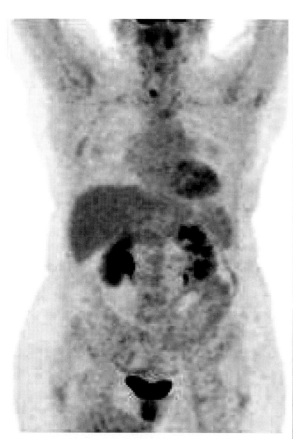

🔳 Thyroid carcinoma after surgery. Tg increasing with negative conventional imaging.

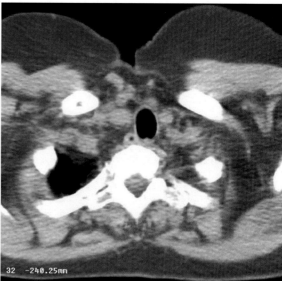

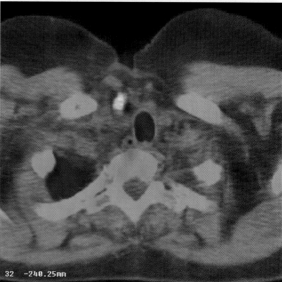

🔳 PET findings

focal FDG increased uptake, suggestive of local relapse

Teaching point

FDG PET is useful in assessing recurrent disease, and being able to identify local relapse as well as nodal and distant lesions.

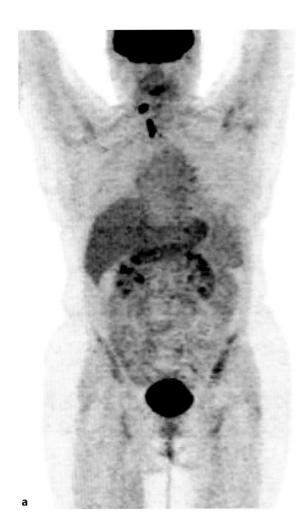

a

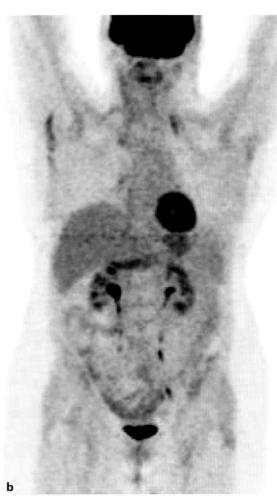

b

Teaching point

PET/CT does not provide any additional
benefit when compared to US and CT for the
initial evaluation of cervical node levels in
patients with papillary thyroid carcinoma.
When 131I scintigraphy is uncertain, PET
is a valid tool to restaging the patient after
therapies.

◘ PET findings

two right laterocervical hypermetabolic lymph
nodes (a). Negative scan after therapy (b)

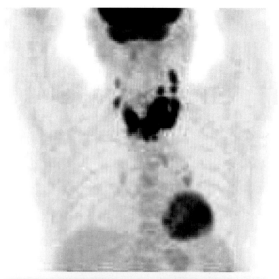

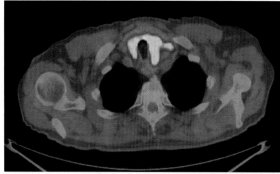

◘ PET findings

diffuse FDG increased uptake at enlarged thyroid and at lymph nodes. At biopsy thyroid lymphoma

Teaching point

FDG PET cannot provide a pathologic diagnosis, but is useful to evaluate the extent of the disease, even in rare situations such as a thyroid lymphoma.

Subject Index